Mozart and the Whale

An Asperger's Love Story

Jerry & Mary Newport
with Johnny Dodd

A TOUCHSTONE BOOK
New York London Toronto Sydney

TOUCHSTONE
Rockefeller Center
1230 Avenue of the Americas
New York, NY 10020

This is a work of nonfiction, however, certain names and identifying
characteristics have been changed.

TOUCHSTONE and colophon are registered trademarks
of Simon & Schuster, Inc.

For information about special discounts for bulk purchases,
please contact Simon & Schuster Special Sales at 1-800-456-6798
or business@simonandschuster.com.

Designed by Elliott Beard

Manufactured in the United States of America

10 9 8 7 6 5 4 3 2 1

Library of Congress Cataloging-in-Publication Data

Newport, Jerry.
    Mozart and the whale : an Asperger's love story / Jerry & Mary Newport,
with Johnny Dodd.
        p. cm.
        1. Newport, Jerry—Health. 2. Newport, Mary—Health. 3. Asperger's
syndrome—Patients—Biography. 4. Husband and wife. I. Newport, Mary.
II. Dodd, Johnny, 1963– III. Title.
    RC553.A88.N59 2007
    362.196'8588320092—dc22
    [B]
                                                            2006050148

ISBN–13: 978-0-7432-7282-7
ISBN–10:   0-7432-7282-X

To You, the reader.
—from Mary and Jerry

To Tex and Miss Ella, my two little comets.
Long may you burn brightly.
—from Johnny Dodd

PROLOGUE

The journey you're about to embark on over the next few hundred pages is, at its heart, a story of love. Our odyssey, like that taken by many others, follows a circuitous route made all the more difficult because we both have Asperger's syndrome. Where normal-brained lovers might encounter speed bumps, we got mired in deep ditches. When others with a different neurological wiring might glimpse a few storm clouds on the horizon, we saw nothing but darkness. The littlest things tore us apart.

This is the story about what happens when two people with Asperger's fall in love. We had to find our own way. We had no road maps to follow and precious few guidebooks to instruct us on what to do once we arrived. Time and time again, we stumbled and fell, then picked ourselves up, convincing ourselves that we'd learned our lesson and wouldn't make the same mistake twice. And then, just when we thought we'd gotten it right, we fell again and again. Love, we quickly learned, wasn't for the weak of heart.

But the funny thing was, neither one of us would trade away any of the heartache and headaches we experienced along the way.

Why? Because the journey we endured not only taught us precious mysteries about one another, it gave us priceless insight into ourselves—far better than any therapist or counselor ever could. We both learned that just because our heads weren't naturally wired for love, it didn't mean our hearts weren't. And it certainly didn't mean we couldn't learn to love. Our tumultuous journey taught us that the first step toward attracting a loving partner is simply to find a way to love yourself. Exactly how you do that is up to you, but one thing's for certain: if you can't love yourself, how can you expect anyone else to?

Our story is hardly unique. There are plenty of children, teens, and adults out there who feel as hopelessly *different* and *unlovable* as we did, who have resigned themselves to believing that they're doomed to live out life without ever feeling like a single person can accept them for who they really are. Our one hope is that people with Asperger's—along with their parents, friends, and caregivers—will recognize the difficulties that come with relationships so they can troubleshoot them rather than walk away from them in defeat. Because people with Asperger's can have great relationships. We can experience love in magical ways that our normal-brained brothers and sisters can never know or understand. Love can lift you higher than you ever thought possible and connect you to the world in a way you can never know until you've experienced it.

Once you taste it, you'll never settle for anything less.

CHAPTER ONE

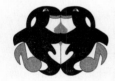The sleeping pills should have kicked in hours ago. I swallowed somewhere close to sixty of them, praying they'd take me away from everything my life had become. I'd thought it all out, all the details. In the event my body wasn't discovered for several days, I'd written a little note, poured out a couple of pounds' worth of seed for my birds, then pulled the curtain closed around my bed, and curled up with Mrs. Willy, my giant stuffed whale. On the other side of the curtain, out by the sliding glass door caked with dirt that rumbled from the Sunday afternoon traffic, my birds sat quietly, staring out into the smog.

I had a hunch they knew.

It hadn't been a good day. In fact, as someone who had endured a lifetime of bad days, the past two years were a new, dismal low. Just when it looked like life was on the verge of being worth living, everything slipped away and turned to shit. Mary was gone and she wasn't coming back. Her birthday was yesterday. I shut my eyes and waited for something to happen. All I knew is that I didn't want to spend the rest of my life alone. Not quite sure why it was taking so long. Certainly seemed like that many pills would do the trick. For an instant, I started to obsess about the number sixty, mulling over what an interesting number it is and how I never imagined I'd die because of it. Sixty is the product of 2 times 2 times 3 times 5. Sixty is the number of degrees of arc covered by the side of a hexagon inscribed inside a circle. Each side equals the radius, and the hexagon is made of six equilateral triangles linked together. Fold them all outside and you get six more, forming a total of twelve, which makes a Star of David with one equilateral triangle for each tribe of Israel. . . . After a few moments, however, I realized I wasn't in the mood to do any calculations or even to think about numbers. The room began to grow quiet, the traffic a bit fainter. I wondered if I was slipping away.

Lying there, I tried not to remember. A lot of good that was doing. It took me my entire life to find Mary, and now she'd gone away. After only five years of marriage, we crashed and burned. She moved back to Tucson and I'm stuck here. A couple of months ago, it looked like maybe we'd get back together, but it didn't last. Don't know why I let myself get my hopes up like that. It just wasn't meant to be. At least not now. But once upon a time it certainly was. . . .

I still remember that Halloween party I'd organized, the one where I first met Mary Meinel. The year was 1993, which happens to be the sum of the squares of 43 and 12. When you add those two numbers up, you get 55, which is the year Mary was born—1955. The day we met was the 289th day of the year, a perfect square of 17. The number 17 is also unique because it's a prime number and you can inscribe a seventeen-sided figure inside a circle, which is rare.

I'd spent weeks trying to construct a whale costume out of garbage bags and paper. The results were laughably pathetic. Strips of newspaper and bits of chicken wire dangled from its side. It resembled a carcass. I ended up dragging it around the party behind me like a deflated blimp. But my costume also reminded me of how magical AGUA was. Because as ridiculous as my costume looked, everybody complimented me on it. They seemed to understand what I was trying to create, and they were proud of me for even attempting such a feat. This kind of unconditional support—whether one succeeded or not—turned out to be one of my favorite parts of AGUA.

I got my first glimpse of Mary as I stood in a hallway, waiting to use the bathroom. My bladder felt on the verge of exploding. Mary opened the restroom door, walked out, and the first thing that hit me was her lavender lace dress. Months before, she'd taken a disposable razor to her head and shaved off her hair. Of course, I didn't know that at the time because she'd pulled this crazy-looking Mozart wig down over her scalp. A cluster of powder white locks dangled and danced around her shoulders. Mary had disappeared into the living room by the time I finally ventured out of the bathroom. She was chatting with some other members of my group. I watched her for a little while, amazed at how she lit up the room. I'd never seen anything like it. When I finally summoned up enough courage to introduce myself, the first words out of my mouth were: "When were you born?"

A smile tiptoed across her face. "March 6, 1955," she replied.

It didn't take me long to come up with the answer—roughly the same length of time required to inhale. "March 6, 1955, was a Sunday," I shouted excitedly. "That's one hundred and nineteen years after the day they ended the siege of the Alamo, which was on March 6, 1836."

Mary clapped her hands together. "That's cool," she giggled. "I guess you're a savant, too?"

That voice of hers. I'd never heard anything quite like it. The sound of it was so undeniably feminine. Definitely the voice of a woman—as opposed to what I was used to hearing at these support group meetings. Half of the women who attended these

gatherings were autistic in name only. Desperate to fit in somewhere, they masqueraded as one of us. They stuck out like Jane
Goodall sitting in the jungle, hanging out with the chimps. Yet all
Mary had to do was open her mouth and you knew she was different. Her words, the way she strung them together, possessed that
unmistakable ring of someone who actually enjoyed listening to
what another person had to say.

Mary's strange habit of finding another person interesting was a
rare trait for someone with Asperger's, a neurological disorder that
tends to lock people in their own private, hermetically sealed universe. I've spent my entire life trying to understand this strange, often
lonely dimension. And whenever some normal-brained person asks
me to describe my condition, I use this analogy: Imagine "normal"
as pure water. Now try to picture autism as whiskey. Asperger's falls
somewhere in between the two. Compared to autism, children with
Asperger's syndrome usually learn to speak at the appropriate age,
though the way they say things may not necessarily sound like other
kids. They also learn self-help skills, such as how to tie their shoes
and brush their teeth, at the same time other kids do. Many of us
with Asperger's remain undiagnosed because we discover a way to
make a living by capitalizing upon our interests and are forgiven for
being a little "off."

This "off-ness" is strongest in areas of social communication.
Those of us with Asperger's can be smart, do well in school, and
maintain a job while also being incredibly thickheaded socially.
For instance, most guys wouldn't ask a girl out more than three
times before getting the hint that she wasn't interested. My record
was fourteen times, a feat that drove one unlucky young woman
to drop the college mathematics class we shared. Men with Asperger's syndrome (and some studies estimate the male-to-female
ratio is 4:1) tend either never to summon up the courage to date at
all or fanatically pursue a person beyond reason. They believe that

their interest and devotion will eventually win her over. It rarely does.

In addition to possessing an average to above-average intelligence, those with Asperger's are often fixated on narrow, intense interests. Conversing with an Aspie can quickly prove frustrating, as he tirelessly attempts to steer a conversation back to his specific area of interest, no matter what others want to discuss. They also tend to take things literally and are oblivious to subtle physical and verbal cues. Their social deficits are often extreme: They either speak too loudly or in a barely audible whisper. They either make too much eye contact or none at all. In other words, when it comes to dealing with people, those of us dwelling on Planet Asperger's just don't get it.

A few weeks after that first meeting with Mary, I was shocked, bewildered, and amazed when she telephoned to ask me a question I hadn't heard in decades: "Do you think we could go out sometime?" A few days later, we hopped a city bus to the Los Angeles County Zoo. I wanted to pinch myself during that first afternoon we spent together, walking among the caged animals. Never in my life had I felt so at ease with another human being, let alone a woman.

Long ago, I'd resigned myself to the unpleasant fact that I'd probably spend the rest of my life alone. The prospect made me so sad that just thinking about it could instantly transform me into a grouch. I'd spent a portion of just about every single day of my life since college daydreaming about how it would feel to fall in love with a woman—the kind of love you read about in grocery store romance paperbacks or see in the movies, where two people skip through a field of clover, laughing and holding hands. But I was desperate and so tired of feeling alone, so tired of wondering why I'd always felt like I had this invisible wall encircling me, preventing me from connecting with another human being.

Mary changed all that. She turned my solar system upside down and shook it until all the planets tumbled out. By the time we embarked on our second date, it was clear that nothing in my life would ever be the same. From then on, I actually began to believe that I'd stumbled upon the one woman in existence with whom I could spend my life. That happened on the 344th day of the year, which fell on Friday, December 10, 1993. Mary was thirty-eight years old. I was forty-five. We'd known each other fifty-five days, which I thought was appropriate because 1955 was the year Mary was born. Even more amazing is if you take the number 55 and multiply it by how many hours are in a day, 24, you end up with 1,320. That just happens to be the number of feet in a quarter mile. My all-time favorite track event in high school was the quarter mile.

Our date started off at the monthly meeting of the West L.A. Bird Club. I was a member. Mary wasn't. But after we recovered from the shock of learning that we both owned cockatiels, it seemed like the perfect place to meet. For years, when neither of us had anyone to turn to, these ridiculously expressive, loyal creatures served as our only friends. They always looked concerned when you stepped out your front door and excited whenever you returned home.

After the bird club gathering broke up, we caught a bus that took us across town to my hopelessly cluttered apartment in Santa Monica. The nighttime air felt out of place for December. It was warm. Then again, maybe it was just my jittery nerves that made the earth seem hotter. Either way, standing this close to an actual female set my mind whirring into overdrive. Decades had lapsed since anything so intimate, so wonderful, seemed on the verge of unfolding. We stood by the front door and I fumbled for my keys. Okay, Jerry, what's it gonna be? Should you ask her to come inside? Then what? Maybe see if she wants to sit on your dirty sofa? Maybe chat her up a bit? Then make your move. Then try to kiss her. . . . It just might work.

The voices in my head were making me dizzy. "I've got an

idea," I blurted out, shoving my keys back into my pocket. "Let's take a walk down to the bluffs. There's something there I think you might enjoy seeing."

"Let's go." Mary laughed. Her lips curled up into the most perfect smile I'd ever seen. Each time she flashed it, my heart beat crazily.

And so, the two of us began our trek down the street to the park, perched up high above the Pacific Ocean. We'd only taken a few steps when I suddenly noticed something. Never in my life, especially not during any date I'd ever endured, had I felt so alive, so absolutely at ease with another person and with myself, so unconcerned with hiding the universe brewing deep inside of me. As Mary and I strolled down Montana Avenue, I suddenly felt as though I'd spent my entire life locked inside a tiny prison cell and in the blink of an eye the walls of my cell had vanished. The sensation of freedom to just be me was dizzying, intoxicating. No longer did I have to pretend to be someone other than who I was, someone who the rest of the world would call normal.

After a few minutes, we came upon a beautifully restored '57 Corvette parked in front of a dry cleaner. The light from a nearby streetlight shimmered off the vehicle's spotless white body. Mary and I stood there admiring it, and before I knew it I was watching the streetlight's glow bouncing off the Corvette's hood, setting Mary's strawberry-tinted wig ablaze. All at once, a domino-like chain of thoughts exploded inside my head. This can't be happening to me. It's all too perfect. Women like Mary aren't interested in guys like me. A voice instructed me to start running and not look back, but I made a decision to ignore it and gently lifted my foot and tapped it against the Corvette's license plate. Mary quickly glanced down at the jumble of numbers and letters on the plate, then looked at me quizzically.

"You want me to do the license plate for you?" I asked.

"Go for it," she laughed, clapping her hands together in anticipation.

"2VoR013," I announced, then quickly plucked the numbers out of the string—20013. My mind began doing what it had done for just about as long as I could remember; it churned out connections and relationships between the various digits. "Hmmm, you know, 20013 is a really fascinating number," I explained.

"Why?" Mary asked. "What makes it so special?"

"Because its prime factors are 3, 7, and 953," I said. "So if you get a 21 in blackjack 953 times, you win enough to pay for the Corvette."

By this point, we've resumed our trek down the sidewalk. Even though I'm not looking at Mary, I can tell she's staring at me. The pressure from her doelike eyes felt like it was burning a hole right through me. I didn't dare look into them. I had a lot of trouble with that. I always had. Gazing into someone's eyes—even for a brief instant—was like standing on the ledge of a skyscraper and peering down into the emptiness below. It petrified me, thinking that I was going to tumble into the abyss. That was why I didn't bother looking at her. I knew she understood. So I just kept walking, running the license plate through my head, over and over again like it was some sort of numerical mantra.

"20013 ... 20013 ... 20013," I mumbled. "Did you know October 17, 1955, was the 20,013th day of this century?"

"Cool." Mary laughed. There was something magical about her voice and how it rumbled up from deep within her throat. Just listening to it caused my cheeks to get all splotchy. I felt like I might be on the verge of hyperventilating. Up ahead of us, I spotted a battered old Saab with a parking ticket on the windshield. The license plate jumped out at me.

"2BYN467 ... 2467 is a prime number," I explained, wondering if maybe I might be overdoing it with all my number tricks. "Did you know if you change 2467 into a binary number, you end up with 100110100011?" I don't bother waiting for Mary to respond. I'm on a roll now. Sparks are practically leaping off my brain. There's no turning back. Farther up ahead, I spot the plate on a Toyota 4Runner. "32908 ... that's my father's birthday—3–29–08,"

I said excitedly, pausing to take a quick breath. "That's also the birthday of Man o' War in 1917, and one day before the birthday of Secretariat in 1970 ... Actually, Secretariat was born at 12:15 a.m. on the thirtieth, in Virginia, eastern time. So he was really born on the twenty-ninth California time."

Shut up, Jerry. That was what I heard inside my head—that all-too-familiar voice telling me to stop all this nonsense before it's too late, before I convinced this truly beautiful woman walking beside me that I was an absolute lunatic. I felt ridiculous. Why on earth did I allow the numbers to do that to me? How could I allow myself to get carried away?

"I'm sorry," I told her. "I didn't mean to go on like that."

Out of the corner of my eye, I sneaked a peek at Mary's face. The expression I expected to find was one of extreme uncertainty, perhaps even revulsion. But when it hit me that she had an ear-to-ear grin plastered on her face, my mouth dropped open.

"You gotta be kidding me." She giggled. "Don't apologize. And don't ever stop. I love it. The universe is made up of numbers."

"Exactly!" I shouted, floored by the unthinkable notion that I'd found a woman who understood. And Mary truly understood. Every speck of matter in the universe, every single solitary thing in it, was constructed from atoms, all of which are fashioned out of various quantities of particles. Once you begin comparing these quantities, a never-ending array of patterns begins to surface. When I looked at a number that was exactly what happened— patterns, relationships, associations emerged and blossomed like flowers. People like Mary, who compose symphonies and paint pictures, experience those sorts of revelations with colors and music. I do it with numbers. For nearly as long as I can remember, numbers have been the single thing I could always relate to, the only phenomena in the world that possessed a sense of order that felt truly reassuring and comforting.

Numbers were all I had.

As we walked, I began to mull over my numerical fixation. And then it happened. Mary was actually grasping my hand. I can't say for sure when she grabbed it. All I knew was that our fingers were entwined and the warm flesh of our soft palms was pressed together. Such a glorious feeling. Nearly two decades had passed since the last time it had happened, when I was in college. Back then, I had plenty of dates. My strategy, although pathetically desperate, was brilliantly simple. I'd hang out in the library. Whenever I spotted a girl with her nose buried in a book, I'd saunter over and begin chatting her up. I've always been something of a generalist, able to spout off an endless array of facts and figures on just about every subject under the sun. Before long, I usually convinced my female targets that I was bright, witty, and—most important—a regular guy. That was the most important thing for me. By the time I exited the library, I'd usually be clutching the woman's phone number on a scrap of paper. A few days later, we'd go out on a date. Then, without fail, she'd realize the truth—she'd been hoodwinked. There was something just not right with me. Sometimes it was worse. They never returned my calls.

Not that I blamed them for writing me off. I was already beginning to do the same thing myself. I just didn't want to admit it. Nevertheless, all my dates became nothing more than excruciating trials of insecurity. The drama unfolding inside my head so consumed me that I rarely paid much attention to my date. All I wanted was for her to think of me as normal. I was obsessed with it. Whenever my date would begin telling me things like where she went to high school, what she was studying, and what she imagined herself doing in the future, I'd never hear a word she said. Instead, I'd be listening to that voice between my ears, the one that either beat myself up or pumped me full of so much self-doubt that I wanted to crawl into a closet and cry. I'd chide myself: What an idiotic thing to say, Jerry!... You sound like a freak!... I wonder what she thinks of me?... When is she going to realize how strange I really am?

No matter how hard I tried, I could never grasp the subtle expressions that flashed across my dates' faces, emotional cues that might have tipped me off to their impression of me at any given moment. Everyone else always seemed able to pick up on these tips. But for me it felt as though I were staring at a wall of hiero-glyphs. No wonder I dreaded those excruciating moments when I would run out of words and find myself walking my date to the front door of her apartment or sitting beside her on the couch. Those moments were absolutely unbearable. And that was when the voice would always begin whispering: What now, Jerry? You gonna touch her hand? How about a little kiss on the cheek? What about on the lips?

Why did I endure such tortures? For the simple reason that my only sense of self came from others. I only existed when others thought of me. And I was convinced that the only way others would bother to think of me was if I was seen with the type of partner who would make me look worth knowing.

More than ten years had passed since my last real date. Not that anybody who glanced over at Mary and me would have known it. To anyone watching, we were just two people strolling down Montana Avenue, holding hands. It was all so normal, so easy, so natural. I wanted to laugh and cry at the same time.

When we finally arrived at the park, the waves were hurling themselves onto the beach a hundred feet below, out past the six lanes of busy Pacific Coast Highway traffic. I heard thunder off in the distance. Mary stared out at the water until I nudged her gently and pointed at a wooden sculpture I'd wanted her to see, perched on the edge of the crumbling sandstone cliff. Shaped like a giant oval, it was big enough for two people to stand within. Which was exactly why I'd brought her here.

"Oh, wow," Mary shrieked, when she spotted it. "Far out." She threw her arms up into the air like some evangelical preacher suddenly seized by God Almighty. She began laughing hysterically and rocking from side to side. Her giggles hit me with the force of a small tornado.

"What on earth is that?" she shouted. "A nautilus?"

"I think it's supposed to be some sort of fertility symbol." I shrugged while slowly moving into the hollow wooden cavern inside the structure. "Come on," I whispered, holding my hand out for her to grab. "Come on in here with me."

Mary giggled. She looked skeptical, not quite sure what to make of my request. Finally, after what seemed like an eternity, she thrust out her arm and grabbed my hand. Mary was strong and possessed all the grace of a bulldozer. After a few awkward moments spent trying to maneuver herself into the statue's center, I finally decided to yank her inside, up into my arms. For a few moments, we balanced ourselves and gazed out over the churning, frothing waters of the Pacific. Salt from the waves mixed with the night air and drifted upward, coating our faces. I sucked the dampness into my mouth, down my throat, then coaxed myself into peering deep into Mary's eyes. A pulse of dizziness hit me, but I manage to calm myself.

"I wanted our first kiss to be here," I told her.

All Mary did was smile. She let me pull her close and press my lips up against hers. I knew my technique must be laughable, but amazingly I didn't dwell on it. And for the first time in my life, a kiss felt unmistakably natural. For once, I wasn't caught up obsessing that I was invading someone's territory.

Then, before I knew it, we were walking back to my apartment. All the way there, I wondered what she'd think of my place. To call it a pigsty would be an insult to pigs. It was a true cesspool, filled with snowdriftlike stacks of junk mail, old newspapers, and magazines, notes I'd scrawled at various autism conferences, rough manuscripts of children's stories and poems, letters to editors of local papers, and political fliers from a volunteer stint I did with Bill Clinton's 1992 presidential campaign. On more than one occasion I'd set out to tidy up the place, but I couldn't quite pull it off. Every time I attempted to toss something into the trash, a horribly uneasy, anxious feeling descended upon me. It wasn't so much that I feared I'd someday need the item; I just couldn't stand the loss of order and control that came with throwing it out. On several occasions, I packed up the entire mess and moved from one apartment to the next, then went for months before unpacking. Sure, my place was a wretched mess, but there wasn't a single scrap of paper in the place that I couldn't find if I needed to.

The moment we walked inside, I kept glancing at Mary's face. I was looking for blatant, telltale signs of revulsion or queasiness on her part—a sneer, a scowl, rolled eyes, or a muffled gasp. Part of having Asperger's meant I was a pathetic judge of facial expression. Even if I saw something, I doubted I'd know how to interpret it.

Miraculously, my mess didn't appear to bother her. We collapsed onto my filthy sofa and began chatting about our birds. I was enjoying the conversation so much that I never had time to browbeat myself. The next thing I knew, we were making out like I'd always dreamed about doing with a real woman.

But something was different. I didn't feel like an invader. If I didn't know better, I'd swear she wanted *this* to happen. Yet, suddenly, without any warning, Mary stopped in mid-kiss. She closed her eyes, stretched her arms up into the air, and yawned.

She's bored, Jerry. She wants to go home now. You blew it. The voice continued, but I commanded it to shut the hell up.

"Maybe we ought to hop into bed," I stammered, shocked by my bravado.

"That," Mary replied, "would be nice."

A few minutes later, we were snuggling together on the bird-eaten brown blanket atop my bed. The sensations from her velvetlike skin pressed against mine nearly overloaded my neural circuitry. One moment it resembled a blowtorch, the next, absolute bliss. I was on the verge of something I couldn't understand, something I didn't have a name for, and for the first time in my life that seemed just fine. Wave after wave of dizziness washed over me. I couldn't speak. All I could do was lie there pathetically and stare up into the ceiling.

"Uhhhh," I mumbled, "I don't have any protection. . . . I wasn't expecting anything like this to happen."

Mary leaned over toward me and slowly opened her eyes. She looked half asleep. "That's okay," she cooed, snuggling up next to me, sliding her willow-like legs beneath mine. "We don't have to do anything. Isn't it wonderful just to be able to lie here together?"

So that's what we did. We just lay there for I don't know how long. Why would I? Time stopped. We held hands. We did not speak. An air of quiet and calm hung over the room like a soft blanket. The only sound came from the pounding of our hearts, mixed with the occasional swallow. For that brief instant, I felt so calm, comfortable, and in control. Even the voice in my head was quiet, too. Or close to it. I heard it whisper: So this is what it feels like? So this is love?

After awhile, the sounds of something moving could be heard from a darkened, cobwebbed corner of my bedroom. My four cockatiels—Pagliacci and his wife, Caruso, along with their two children, Cockatiel Dundee and Isadora Duncan—had finally summoned up the courage to investigate the strange goings-on in my bed. One by one, they flapped their wings, soared through the blackness, and landed on a nearby curtain rod, just above our heads. Mary opened her eyes and smiled her perfect smile that made my heart tap-dance. They had no idea what to make of the scene unfolding beneath them. I'd never brought a woman into my bedroom before. I couldn't even remember the last time I'd ever even invited another human being into my apartment. The four birds peered down at us with curious looks of concern in their tiny eyes. Pagliacci rocked his tiny head up and down in the air excitedly, then opened his beak and began squawking. Within seconds, the rest of his brood nodded their heads in agreement and began dancing a little jig, their tiny claws clattering as they moved back and forth along the curtain rod.

"If I didn't know better," I told Mary, "I'd have to say they approve of you."

Twenty weeks after that magical night, I stood beneath the gnarled umbrella-like branches of a tired old fig tree and asked Mary to be my wife. The way I saw it, I couldn't have chosen a more auspicious time and place to propose. After all, April 30, 1994, was the 120th day of the year. It also happened to be one week prior to the 120th Kentucky Derby. As numerical fate would have it, that very fig tree we stood beneath first sprouted from the soil on the same year as the running of the first Kentucky Derby. Even more intriguing was that April 30 marked the 28th week since I'd first met Mary at that costume party. Twenty-eight is a big number for me—my absolute favorite. How could it not be? After all, when you add up all the numbers that divide into it, you get 28. The same thing happens when you add up all the integers from 1 to 7. You get 28. But the numerical parallels didn't stop there. The more I pondered the situation, the more everything seemed to fit together like a puzzle. Mary's mother was born 28 Saturdays before her father, and my birthday is sandwiched exactly in the middle of both of theirs—14 weeks after her mother's and 14 weeks before her father's. The day I proposed to Mary happened to be a Saturday. And then there's that business about the number 65—the concrete fence that surrounded our fig tree consisted of 65 pillars and Mary's birth occurred on the 65th day of 1955. For a numbers guy like me, it just doesn't get any numerically purer than that. Everything fit together so neatly, so perfectly. All the various components just seemed to belong.

And so I took Mary's big hand in mine and asked, "Will you be my wife?" I looked into her eyes, hidden by the synthetic bangs of her nut-brown wig, each strand shimmering in the sunlight. "I will," she replied. We wrapped our arms around each other and I shut my eyes and rested my cheek on her shoulder. I felt as though I was embracing a lifetime of hopes and dreams. I was excited, relieved, and petrified. All at once, everything I'd ever wanted in life was positioned right here between my arms, but all I'd ever expected out of life was disappointment and rejection. The moment was so perfect I thought I might pass out.

Years before, I promised myself that if I ever could find a woman who truly loved me, all I'd need to do was spend a single day with her. That's all it would take to make me happy for the rest of my life—just the memory of our single, perfect day together. But there I was on the verge of something truly unthinkable—getting to live out the rest of my life with the woman of my dreams, a woman who loved me just as much as I loved her. Before I met Mary, I'd have told you the odds of such an occurrence were too great for even a numbers guy like me to calculate. But statistical anomalies do happen. Steep odds can be beaten. And for the first time in my sad life, I'd done just that. I'd finally trumped the odds. I'd won the lottery without even purchasing a ticket.

I opened my eyes and realized I wasn't dead. I was merely alone, just like I've been my entire life. It was after midnight. I felt groggy and stupid. Fumbling for the phone, I dialed the number of my supervisor at the medical department at UCLA, where I'd been hired four years before by people with good intentions. But in between my alienating the staff and their dumbing down my workload, I'd become a vastly overpaid gofer. And if it wasn't for my "condition," I would have been fired years ago.

"I'm not feeling well," I mumbled. "I won't be coming in tomorrow." I dropped my head back onto the pillow and hugged

Mrs. Willy. I couldn't understand why I was still alive. Nearly sixty sleeping pills and it hadn't done a thing. Good lord, I'd heard of people going out with much less than that. After awhile, a thought that could only be described as comforting percolated up inside my head. Maybe you're not supposed to die just yet.

For the next ten minutes, I pondered that peculiar riddle, staring up at the ceiling until my eyelids got too heavy to hold open. Maybe there's a reason why you're still here, I heard the voice mumble.

Maybe it's time to start finding out why.

TUCSON, ARIZONA
OCTOBER 1999

It certainly seemed like a feasible plan. First, I'd take the pills. Next, I'd duct tape the garbage bag over my head. Then, just to play it safe, I'd slit my wrists with a razor. I positioned a trash can on both sides of my bed to ensure I didn't make too much of a mess. I had a handful of suicide attempts under my belt, so I pretty much had it all figured out. The trick was really all in the way you slit your wrists. Most people just don't slice correctly. You need to sever the arteries and the only way to do that is by pressing the razor deep into your wrist, an inch or two south of the veins. It really hurts when you do that. But if you don't do it correctly, then all you do is mess up the ligaments in your wrists. Not good. Because not only do you continue living, but you can never use your hands again. I definitely didn't want that. All I wanted was to become nothing, which I had a hunch was what happened when you die. Just a whole lot of sweet nothing.

I'd been thinking about killing myself for the past month. Every day, when I'd walked down the dusty streets of the barrio where I lived in Tucson, on my way to the grocery, I passed a cryptic billboard. It read, YOU ARE NOT INDISPENSABLE. I never could figure out what it was an ad for, but I felt like it had been written just for me. All day long, I'd think about that billboard, and it never failed to remind me of what a mess I'd made of everything between the two of us. It certainly wasn't entirely my fault, but lately the clouds had lifted just enough so that I'd begun to understand my role in things. I'd come so close to success, so close to finding real love that it hurt. And now all I had to show for our time together was a big empty hole in my chest where my heart used to be.

Jerry stopped by a few days ago. He drove out from Los Angeles to pick up the birds. I don't think he understood what I was intending to do. I needed him to take them away from here. I was afraid to think what would happen to them when I was gone.

If I'd had to guess, I would have thought that about twenty minutes had passed since I swallowed what was left of my bottle of antipsychotic medication. Wasn't too sure exactly how many were in there, but it definitely should have been enough to anesthetize me so I could do what needed to be done with the razor. When I felt the familiar grogginess settle in, I pulled the garbage bag over my head, then wrapped a strip of duct tape around my neck and just sat there on the edge of my bed. The rumble of the trucks roaring in and out of the bottling plant next door caused my bed to shudder. Or maybe it was just my nerves.

After a few minutes, the claustrophobia hit me. I tried to pretend it wasn't happening by taking a few deep breaths, but that wasn't easy inside a garbage bag. Then I tried to press the razor against my left wrist. It felt hopelessly awkward since I couldn't see anything. Should have thought of that, Mary, I scolded myself. And that was when I started to have second thoughts about my foolproof way out. It was the middle of a hot afternoon, in the middle of the week, in the middle of the month, and I suddenly felt stupid and hopelessly alone inside this old house, with a plastic bag taped over my head. My heart began pounding. I began to think about things: What were the odds that I'd actually manage to kill myself anyway? After all, I'd read about people cutting off their hands in factories and never managing to bleed to death. I tore the bag off my head. The last thing I wanted was for Jerry to feel guilty if something happened to me here. He deserved better than that. After all, he was my soul mate. That much was clear even on our second date.

That image of us marching along Montana Avenue was tattooed into my memory. I couldn't wash it off, no matter how hard I tried. That was the night all of this craziness started. After that, there was no turning back.

Jerry was anxious. But it was the good kind of anxiousness. Like the way a child gets when he opens his eyes and suddenly realizes it's Christmas morning. I could feel nearly everything going on inside his head without him ever uttering a single word. Autistics can sometimes do that with each other. It's an intuitive thing. We can sense in a way that sometimes extends far beyond words. Although God knows how many times I would have been content to rely solely on words, like a normal-brained person. Perhaps we swap one form of communication for another more mysterious, less understood one? But throw us into a room filled with people whose brains function in a so-called normal, predictable way, and we're hard-pressed to grasp even the most basic display of emotion. The normal world has the same problem with us. To them, we appear distant, alien, and hopelessly detached, as if trapped behind an invisible force field.

I seriously doubted that anyone who spotted us on that December evening would have had the slightest idea about the mind-blowing significance of that night. To any onlooker, we were just two odd-looking middle-aged people out for a walk, staring at license plates and laughing.

Jerry was a sight to behold. I'd never seen anything like him, especially on a date when most guys were usually going out of their way trying to make a good impression. By that point in our lives, I think we were both getting awfully tired of worrying about impressions. I know I was. So I didn't put a lot of thought into the fact that he showed up in the uniform he wore for his courier job—a spiffy white pressed shirt with his name stitched in cursive blue thread over his left breast pocket. Jerry had a strawlike mop of hair on his head. Just one look at his coif and I could tell he'd styled with his fingers. It was a look I found attractive, since I've always been a sucker for that tousled boyish look, especially on a big man like Jerry.

Yet what truly attracted me to him was what lay deep underneath all that messed-up hair. I glimpsed it the first time we met. It was that part of him that he'd kept hidden away for all those years and was only now beginning to feel comfortable exposing to others. He possessed a mysterious mixture of boy and man. Jerry could stare at an animal and react with the wide-eyed, goofy wonder of a child. Then, the next thing you knew, he uttered something so profound you found yourself pondering it for weeks.

But more than anything else, I loved to listen to him carry on about numbers. And that night on our second date, when the two of us were wandering down Montana Avenue, I didn't want him to stop because of how happy he appeared finally to be sharing his world with someone. Jerry wove webs out of numbers. He glimpsed relationships among them that few people can fathom. How on earth he could glimpse the common thread that stretches between one number and the next, I hadn't a clue. But then, I didn't really have to—just as the average person doesn't have to know a thing about music theory in order to be blown away by the staggering beauty of Mozart's creations. All one had to do was listen to Jerry ramble about his numerical epiphanies to know you were in the presence of a gifted person.

When Jerry finally got it in his head to kiss me, the two of us were shaking like leaves. We both had so many strange feelings, generated by years' worth of frustration, loneliness, and empty hope, that one day we'd find someone with whom we could feel whole and normal. Jerry hadn't been with too many women. That was pretty clear. In contrast, I'd been around the block so many times I needed new tires. Although I'd endured many long stretches of celibacy, back during my tie-dyed hippie days, I bedded plenty of men. Yet all I really wanted was for one of them to see something inside of me that I'd never been able to find myself. Of course, they never did. So I drifted from one guy to the next, always thinking my latest conquest would be my knight, the one who would tell me he loved me, who'd whisper in my ear that I wasn't the freak everyone told me I was.

For as long as I could remember, I wondered why the world seemed so revolted by me, so repulsed. Eventually, I stopped searching for answers and resigned myself to the wretched hand I'd been dealt. If the world wanted me to be a freak, then that was just what I'd be—the world's biggest, most revolting freak. My family treated me as though I'd arrived here in a spaceship from some distant planet. To nearly everyone I encountered as a child, I seemed hopelessly off. So I coped the best I could, spending most of my time either laughing hysterically while rocking uncontrollably, or possessed by angry rages that reduced me to a shrieking pint-sized psychopath. Sometimes I'd sit for hours at a stretch, lost in silent, solitary contemplation. On a good day, I could usually be found in the backyard with my arms outstretched, peering up into the heavens, spinning furiously around and around in the grass, lost in the dizzying sensations, laughing like a maniac until I collapsed.

Everything I've written here about my past is the truth as I remember it, pieced together through the haze of my memory. But memories can be deceptive, especially when they're stored in a container that's been cracked as many times as mine has. There are days I believe all the words I've written here to be the literal truth. Other times, I realize that everything I recall from my past is simply the reconstructed narrative of how I experience events, rather than how they actually happened. It's no wonder I have such a rough time deciphering the difference between what is real and what is imagined—I've lived a hard life. Part of the time, the road I've taken has led me over mountain peaks, providing me with views so breathtaking I wanted to cry from the sheer ecstasy of it all. At other moments, the journey pulled me through valleys so dark and bleak I yearned to end my life, to be no more.

What I didn't know then, but now have begun to understand, is that I was hardly the only person in my family to suffer from Asperger's. I think we all had it in varying degrees, including my parents. We were a family of hopeless but absolutely brilliant geeks, forever different from the world around us. And through some cosmic genetic joke, I was the most different of all, with a nervous system far too fragile to deal with the chaos of my quirky, wacky family. It wasn't so much that I needed a different set of parents— in fact, if it weren't for them I wouldn't have been blessed with all my wonderful gifts for music and art. But in the best of all worlds, I should have been an only child, allowed to develop in quiet and cloistered seclusion. Instead, I was dropped in the middle of what seemed to be a perpetual war zone and I'm still shell-shocked from the experience.

My parents didn't know what to do with me. Nobody did. They both tried their best to love me, but they were terrified of me. Deep down I've always thought they both believed I was insane, a prospect that seemed to confirm their most dreadful fear—that the gene for madness ran through our family.

By the time I turned fourteen, I'd grown so out of control they packed me up and handed me over to a paranoid Christian cult in Texas. Actually, I was so mixed up at that point, such a neophyte to the topsy-turvy chaos unfolding inside my mind, I was the one who first suggested it. The group's leader preached that Armageddon lurked just around the corner. My older sister, Barbara, had joined up with the group years before. She raved about the camaraderie and sisterly love she'd found there. So my parents believed this cult, known as the Children of God, offered the perfect holding pen for their wayward daughter. After all, it was either that or an institution. And what parent really wants to ship their child off to the funny farm?

They nearly whooped with relief on that afternoon they dropped me off at the group's muddy, remote compound, then roared off down the highway to freedom. They never looked back, probably because they couldn't bear to. But I stood there in the mud watching them anyway, waiting for one of them to glance back at me, longing for them to raise their eyes and try to catch a glimpse of me in the rearview mirror. I ached to see the darks of their pupils. Instead, they both just sat there in the front seat, ramrod straight, peering through the dirty windshield as my father stomped on the accelerator and sped down that muddy dirt road back to the highway.

Maybe that was why I always had such a difficult time with other people's eyes. When I needed them most, they were nowhere to be found. Since then, it seemed like so much of my life had been spent either repulsed or hypnotized by them. In fact, I don't think I ever truly met a pair of eyes that I felt comfortable with until I looked into Jerry's. He wasn't judging me. I could feel it by the way he looked at me. And that was really what I remembered most about our first kiss. Not so much the awkward movement of Jerry's lips, but that look in his eyes. Pure compassion, understanding, and tenderness. Until that day, whenever I summoned the courage to look into the eyes of one of my lovers, all I saw was my blurry mirrored image gazing dumbly back at me, calling out: "Freak ... Monster ... Beast."

No one had ever looked at me the way Jerry did. Not once in my life had I felt anyone truly attempt to see me, to focus his vision squarely on me. Not like Jerry did when we kissed for the first time inside that hollowed-out wooden sculpture. And by the time we walked back to his apartment, I was positively smitten. He seemed to feel the same way, only there was something about

his klutzy approach at unlocking his front door that led me to
believe he had a bad case of butterflies in his stomach. I liked that.
I couldn't remember the last time I'd made someone nervous like
that—nervous in a good kind of way.

Once inside Jerry's place, he took my hand and gently guided
me along a narrow trail he'd cut through the mess. I'm extremely
tough to offend, but the pungent odor of dust mixed with mildew
nearly overwhelmed me. The artifacts from Jerry's world surrounded me—his ancient typewriter on the dining room table; the
black-and-white head from his Willy the Whale costume leaning
against a pile of papers; a broken Zenith television set coated with
an inch of dust. We sat there in silence for a few moments, gazing
out at his private sea of clutter.

"I have trouble throwing things out," he confessed. All I could
do was softly squeeze his hand and smile. I felt his body relax.
Somewhere in another room, I could hear the fluttering of wings.
I told myself they might belong to angels.

"Would you accept me as your husband?" Jerry asked five
months after that night. After years of searching, I'd somehow
stumbled upon another human being who finally understood the
lonely, frustrating world where I'd spent my entire life. Afterward,
we stood there, the two of us, and I looked deep into Jerry's eyes.
For the first time in my life, I didn't detest the reflection I saw staring back at me.

But good things don't last. At least, they seldom seemed to in my
life. Five years later, I'd pushed Jerry away from me and ran. And
now I'd lost more than a friend. I'd thrown away my entire support network. I felt so isolated, I might as well have been sitting
on the moon.

"I need to go to the hospital," I shouted the moment I heard
my housemate walk through the front door. "I popped a bunch of
pills." She walked into my desolate room, stared at me blankly for

a moment, then wandered down the hallway to find the telephone and call a taxi. I tried to stand up, but my head was spinning from all those pills. So I just sat there on the bed and waited and stared dumbly out the broken, barrio-dust-covered window.

"They'll be here in a minute," she announced, sounding concerned over having to make the phone call. A moment later, I felt myself stand upright and stumble uneasily out through the open front door, out into the bright, dusty afternoon. The glare made me shield my eyes. All I wanted to do was sleep as I dreamily watched the cab pull up to the curb. It stopped. I smiled. Couldn't help it. Whenever I spotted a taxi, I thought about Jerry and all the years he'd spent driving one on the streets of San Diego. I pulled open the door, collapsed into the backseat, and closed my eyes. For a brief moment, I tried to imagine Jerry was my driver. I tried to pretend I still felt love for him. But just then, as the cab took me away from there, the only thing I felt was failure.

CHAPTER TWO

In the beginning, I was numerically perfect. Born in a corner room in Little Falls Hospital with a big coal-black number 28 painted on the door, I thought my entrance into this world seemed wonderfully auspicious. With all those uniquely wonderful mathematical properties associated with the number 28, I must have felt the soft stirrings of something magical over the implications of being born in a room with that number painted on the door.

I know precious little about the events surrounding Mary's birth. But I've often wondered about it. Sometimes in my dreams, I've seen myself walking into the hospital room where she's lying in a crib. The room is empty except for us. And I go to her, awkwardly taking her into my arms, studying her face for a few moments, then whispering to her that I think she's perfect just the way she is, reminding her never to believe it when, in the years to come, that feeling will start to hit her and try to convince her that she's anything but.

What I remember most about the early days of my childhood

were the whispers. Most people grow up hearing snippets about all the cute, silly activities they engaged in as newborns—inappropriate spit-ups, incessant drooling, incontinence. Instead, I grew up listening to the family lore about how I pushed away my mother when the nurse placed me in her outstretched arms. It still hurts to think about those first few moments of my life. It conjures up too many memories of the fallout that followed. My mother wanted a teddy bear. She wanted to hug and snuggle. For me, hugs represented a loss of control. They made me feel like I was being squeezed to death by one of those giant deep-sea clams in my brothers' comic books. Hugs caused me to shiver and flinch. As is common with many autistic children, I was a "tactile defensive" baby. I never hugged back. I pushed my mother away whenever she attempted to hold me. She never gave up wanting "contact" with me, but by the time I turned two, she'd tossed in the towel and stopped trying.

The irony was, deep down, I desperately yearned to be touched, to be held. Just not physically.

For just about as long as I can remember, I was an odd duck in a world of swans. Then again, perhaps describing my family as swans might be pushing it. My parents weren't naturals when it came to raising a family. Both had been brought up by foster parents. And even though their childhood and teen years were comfortable, they grew up feeling like a burden to the relatives who raised them. What united them was a deep desire for their three boys to have a real mom and pop. They managed to pull off this feat in the best way they could but felt compelled to constantly remind us of all the sacrifices they were making on our behalf. When I think back to my childhood, it often felt like I was being raised by a mother and father who acquired all their parenting skills by reading a civil service manual. I always wondered why they waited a decade after their marriage before deciding to start a family. They always felt old to me. As a kid, I always wished that I had appeared in their lives when they were still young.

Perhaps it shouldn't be surprising that I felt so out of place, so peculiar as a child. My first true fear was of heights, which made navigating the stairs in our house in Trumansburg, New York, where my father ran a Chevy dealership with his brother, a terrifying ordeal. Eventually, I stumbled upon a technique that took a bit of the edge off. Gripping the banister with all my strength, I'd inch my way down backward, literally moving one step at a time. Cautiously, I'd drop my right foot down onto the step, then slide my left foot down onto the same step. It took me forever to complete my trek, but it was the only way I could stomach the journey.

Then there were those two wildly vivid recurring dreams that I never seemed to be able to shake from my head when I awoke in the morning. In the first one, I was sitting on a wooden bridge as a diesel locomotive barreled toward me, black smoke gushing from its engine. Despite the danger, I didn't move. I just stared at it, resigned to my unpleasant fate. Then, in the nick of time, my brother Jim and my father came running out of nowhere and pushed me out of the way as the train roared past.

In the other dream, I was standing beside a highway when I glimpsed a dog sitting on the white dividing line. In a flash, I was seized by the uncontrollable desire to run my hand across its soft fur. But there was one little catch: a large truck was also roaring its way toward the dog. Despite the realization that if I stepped onto the asphalt I would be flattened, I desperately yearned to give the little fellow a reassuring pat on the head. Then, just as I was about to take that fateful first step toward him, I felt my brother John grab my shirt and yank me back to safety. I can still recall that wonderfully comforting feeling of calm whenever I'd wake up knowing that my brothers cared enough to save me.

The one thing my brother John did was teach me how to speak, although technically his pet crow did the teaching. Shortly after my birth, John discovered the baby bird in our backyard, caught it with his bare hands, and stuck it inside a tiny metal cage that hung beside my crib. After nursing the animal back to health, he taught it a few words and named it Blackie. I spent hours lying there, staring up at this sinister-looking black creature, listening to its shrieks. Thanks to Blackie's tutelage, the first word to roll out of my mouth was *hello*. The utterance of this simple greeting proved to be a pivotal moment in my relationship with my mother. When she heard that first word float out from my lips, she decided that if she couldn't hold me, she could at least reach out and touch me with verbal logic—with words.

Since my only way of experiencing the world was verbally, it's only logical that I began to take things literally, following any and all rules with absolute blind allegiance. The first time this trait revealed itself came during breakfast one morning when my brothers were locked in a heated debate over some topic I couldn't quite understand. My mother spent a few minutes listening to their bickering, then reached her breaking point and shrieked, "If you two don't cut that out this instant, I'm going to walk out the front door and never come back!"

I broke out laughing, unable to fathom what I was hearing. Had she gone insane? Because of our maddening habit of tracking mud through the house, my brothers and I knew that one of the steadfast, unbreakable rules of our house was that the front door was something we opened only for guests. We were a back-door family. That much had been drilled into our heads. Which is why I shouted, "No, Ma, if you're gonna leave, you better use the back door!"

Nobody moved after that. My family just stared at me, no doubt waiting for what I just said to make sense. But it never did. Not to them, at least. So my brothers went back to their breakfasts, quietly wolfing down their oatmeal, looking embarrassed by

the strange nonsense that had just come out of my mouth. Their
reaction frightened me. And it was then I began to understand: I
wasn't like anyone else I'd ever met. I was ... different.

As a child, I never could shake this feeling that my actions and
utterances were strangely out of sync with the world around me,
annoyingly off-key. I began to suspect that something peculiar was
incubating inside of me. Yet I couldn't quite put my finger on it
and, to make matters more frustrating, I couldn't do anything to
make the feeling go away. I felt out of kilter, different. At any given
moment, I believed myself on the verge of saying something so
ridiculous and disconnected from the world around me that I just
knew everybody within earshot was going to stand there and laugh
at me. I lived gripped by the fear that my strangeness was just one
sentence away from being revealed. The older I got, the more it
seemed as if the lights were being dimmed. I sensed a darkness
without a name enveloping me. All I could do was grope for something to hang onto and pray I could prevent myself from falling
into the abyss. Something was beginning to go terribly wrong.

Nothing quite stirred up these early feelings of self-loathing
like Donald Duck. Even though he was only a cartoon character,
I hated him. The way he'd get all flustered, then come unglued to
the point where he'd begin kicking his little webbed feet and flail-
ing his feathered arms, struck too close to home. Donald wasn't
an animated duck. He was a personal attack. On more than one
occasion, I'd watch his angry convulsions up on the massive screen
at the local movie theater and suddenly hear myself whisper a lie
to one of my brothers: "I gotta use the bathroom."

Instead, I wandered out into the lobby, sat on a bench, and
stared intently at the popcorn machine for the next hour or
so—anything to get away from Donald. By the time the Jerry
Lewis feature we'd come to see appeared on the screen, I'd be in
no mood to return to my seat. So I'd just continue sitting there,

trying to drown out Jerry's spastic whining and screaming. I'd
cringe as his awful voice hit my ears, trying to work its way inside
my head, angry that we shared the same first name. When the
feature was over, one of my brothers would appear in the lobby
looking for me, shaking his head, unable to fathom why in God's
name I'd go to the movies, then spend all my time sitting alone
watching corn pop.

I'm a stickler for details. So it's probably not surprising that I can
pinpoint the precise moment my life crumbled and I got my first
real glimpse of that dark thing awakening inside me. It happened
on Thanksgiving of 1952—which my gift for these sorts of things
tells me occurred on November 27. My family and I had been invited to my uncle Bob's house in Trumansburg. I was standing in
his backyard, walking toward a marshy, wooded area at the back
of his property. The autumn sun was sinking below the trees.
My father, brothers, cousins, and uncle ventured off toward the
woods, but I found myself inexplicably preoccupied with a thread
of geese winging their way south up in the darkening sky. I was
lagging behind the group, something I often did. But all at once
everything felt different. I'd never felt quite so . . . separate. Everybody stopped to turn and look at me, plodding through the mud.
Nobody spoke. They just stared. The expression on their faces felt
uncomfortably similar to the one I'd seen my brothers make at the
breakfast table, months earlier—a combination of bewilderment,
amusement, and incredulity.

A few minutes later, we arrived back at Uncle Bob's house.
Everyone was talking and laughing, conversations flowed effortlessly around me. But I felt hopelessly unable to enter into any of
them. In the past, I'd often found this type of social interaction
tough. But the situation in Uncle Bob's living room seemed absolutely insurmountable. I'd become a ghost, completely cut out
of the scene, hopelessly out of sync. When I did manage to speak

and someone interrupted me, I'd get so frustrated and angry that
I'd immediately clam up. Then I'd wander over to another group,
where I'd attempt to jump into their discussion, always at the
wrong moment, always rambling on about some obscure topic
that had been raised minutes before.

That night, after we returned to our house, I stood in the bathroom, studying myself in the mirror, inspecting the reflection of my
face, thinking about everything that had just happened. Strange, I
certainly seemed to look like everyone else. So how come nobody
would pay any attention to me? Why did I feel so separate? For
the first time in my life I couldn't explain my remoteness away by
reminding myself that I was younger than everyone else. As much
as I hated to admit it, even my younger cousins had been more in
tune, more comfortable with the situation in Uncle Bob's house.

And then it dawned on me: I was *different*. There, I'd put my
finger on it. I wasn't like anyone I knew. I wondered if everyone
felt so alone in the world.

By the time my first day of kindergarten rolled around, my burden
had become familiar. Yet it was still as unwieldy as walking around
with a bag of rocks on your back. Trying to keep the load balanced proved horribly difficult. I never quite knew when or how
my burden would shift. Trying to grasp the delicate nuances of
social boundaries quickly proved my biggest problem. At that
time, I didn't have a single friend, other than my brothers. Yet
there was a boy in my class who tolerated me. His name was
Eric. One Saturday afternoon, I walked across town to visit him. I
knocked on the door of his house. No one answered. Just then, I
noticed that my bladder had become uncomfortably full. The next
thing I knew, I was shimmying up the elm tree on the side of his
house and crawling in through an open bedroom window. When
his family arrived home, they found me sitting on the toilet in the
upstairs bathroom. Eric's father informed his stunned family that

he'd drive me back to my house. He put me in the backseat of the family station wagon, started the car, and periodically glanced at me in the rearview mirror all the way back. I couldn't place it back then, but now I understand his eyes were filled with worry. He didn't say a single word.

A few weeks later, I found myself standing outside our house, knocking on the back door. The school bus had just dropped me off. It was getting dark. For some reason, nobody was home yet. I began to worry. One of my parents' commandments was: Thou shalt be inside the house before it gets dark. Or else! Because I never dared violate any rule, no matter how trivial, it only seemed natural to use my lunchbox to shatter the glass in our back door and let myself inside. I was sitting at the kitchen table working on a puzzle when the rest of my family arrived home a few minutes later. My father's face went red when he spotted the shards of glass littering the floor. He didn't know what the hell to make of my weird behavior. His eyes were filled with that same look of fear and worry that I'd glimpsed in the rearview mirror of Eric's family station wagon.

In June 1954, when I was six, my father's career as a car salesman and his marriage to my mother were spiraling downward. He'd had a falling-out with his brother and, because of the dark mood at our house, there was talk of me and my brothers being shipped off to live with a relative who worked as a Methodist minister. Instead, our father decided to take a teaching job at a high school in Islip, New York, on Long Island. I helped pack our belongings into the moving van, which I kept thinking was a "moving band," and spent the next twelve hours waiting for the music to start.

It never did, of course. But not long afterward I began hearing a different type of music—numbers. It happened one night at a railroad crossing. My brothers and I were sitting in the backseat of our Oldsmobile, throwing elbows. My father, either hoping to prevent any further bruising or because he'd lost his mind, began counting the freight cars out loud as they rumbled past us. I looked up and was suddenly amazed to see that each time another railcar shot past us, he'd shout out a number. Suddenly, something exploded inside of me. I already knew how to count, but in that instant numbers made sense. They weren't abstract. They were real. They had meaning. They surrounded me. If I wanted to, I could literally touch them.

I've always believed my brother John spotted something in my face that night in the backseat. He sensed my epiphany. He could feel it. A half hour later, when we arrived home, he took me into his bedroom and showed me his science project, which had netted him a blue ribbon at the regional science fair, consisting of one of those globes with a lightbulb inside of it. He'd poked it full of pinholes and, when he switched on the bulb, all the constellations were visible on the globe's surface. Using the finger he normally used for poking me, he painstakingly traced his way across our galaxy, naming one constellation after another. I couldn't have cared less about the names. All I wanted to do was count the individual stars. I had become a number junkie and, more than anything else, I needed to feed my habit.

My brother wasn't the only person who saw something in me that I didn't or couldn't. We had a neighbor named Lois, who was in eighth grade with my brother John when I was a first grader. I loved to read by then. Lois, who yearned to be a teacher when she grew up, knew of my love for reading and how I enjoyed learning new vocabulary words. My parents often hired her to watch me whenever they'd go out. She'd arrive at the house with a stack of vocabulary flash cards. We'd sit in the kitchen, she'd hold up one card after another, and the two of us would discuss each new word. After awhile, my lack of eye contact started to concern her.

"You need to look at people when you speak to them," Lois explained in her soft voice. I turned my head away as she spoke. And that's when Lois did something that I couldn't remember anyone else ever doing before. She reached out and gently touched my face with her fingers, then turned my head so I was looking directly at her. A split second before, I had seen her hand moving toward my cheek, but I felt powerless to do anything about it. By the time her fingers made contact with my flesh, I braced myself for the inevitable reaction—that all-too-familiar claustrophobic sense of panic. But it never arrived. Her touch didn't bother me because she was doing it for the right reasons.

It was around the time of my first touch that I discovered *Willie the Operatic Whale,* an animated feature about a leviathan who desperately yearned to sing at the New York Metropolitan Opera. The ungainly, earnest Willie affected me. I often pondered Willie's simple, tear-jerking story, which opens when word leaks out about an opera-singing whale who lives at the North Pole. The musical and scientific communities react to the revelation with jeers and disbelief. Not that Willie cares. He just keeps on belting out an aria from *The Barber of Seville* with the passionate abandon of an aquatic Pavarotti. When Professor Tetti Tatti learns of the animal's purported abilities, he becomes fixated on the idea that Willie must have swallowed an opera singer and obviously has him locked up as a prisoner inside his gargantuan belly. Tetti Tatti organizes an expedition, ventures up into the northern latitudes and, despite Willie's best efforts to dissuade him, fires a harpoon into the whale's chest, killing this obviously gifted creature.

Following the death scene, the narrator intones: "Now Willie will never sing at the Met. But don't be too harsh on Tetti Tatti. He just didn't understand. You see, Willie's singing was a miracle, and people aren't used to miracles. . . . But miracles never die. And somewhere in whatever heaven is reserved for creatures of the deep, Willie is still singing."

Since we were devout Presbyterians, I had a difficult time swallowing the concept that Willie was actually hanging out in the heaven I'd been learning about in Sunday school. But this notion of being misunderstood, of not fitting in, of having something so special locked up inside of you, was very real to me. After awhile, I became secretly convinced that the cartoon had been created solely for my enjoyment. And whenever I could quiet my head long enough to drown out the outside world, there were moments when I swore I could hear Willie's rich baritone singing just for me.

Sometime in the autumn of 1955, during my second-grade year, my mother started working as a substitute math teacher. One night after dinner, a piece of paper fell out of her bag in the kitchen. I picked it up and stared at it, confused by what I saw. Nothing added up.

"These are multiplication tables," she explained.

"What's that?" I asked.

A moment later, she'd filled me in on the theory behind multiplication, squares, and square roots.

"Got it." I smiled. "Thanks."

My mother looked at me a bit quizzically, shrugged her shoulders, and smiled wearily.

Not long afterward, on a Sunday afternoon, it happened. My father was seated at the dining room table, performing his monthly calculations for the local Presbyterian church we attended. In front of him sat an old crank calculator, a sheet of paper, and a box filled with offering envelopes from the morning services. His job was to add up the day's take. He'd already scribbled more than two dozen single-digit numbers onto the page and had begun inputting them into the adding machine, pulling down the lever with each new entry.

I walked over to him, glanced at the scrawl of numbers, and picked up his pencil. Then I wrote a number down on a piece of paper and waited for him to finish crunching numbers on the adding machine. Without saying a word, I slid the paper in front of him. My father looked at it for a second, not sure what I was showing him. Then, all at once, his eyes grew enormous.

"How did you do that?" he demanded. Even the family parakeet was staring at me from his cage in the corner of the room.

What's he making such a fuss about? I wondered. It didn't seem like any big deal. I merely looked at a page filled with numbers, added them up inside my head, and spit out the answer. I couldn't explain how I did it. It just happened. The answer came to me as easily and naturally as looking out the kitchen window and identifying the color of the leaves on the elm tree in our backyard.

"Come on, how'd you do that?" he asked me again.

I just stared at him, not quite sure what to say. For as long as I could remember, I'd yearned for this sort of attention. But now that I was getting it, it seemed a bit bewildering, confusing, negative. I wanted to be praised for all the things other people got praised for—hitting a baseball, telling a funny joke. Not for doing some weird trick with numbers that I couldn't quite explain. Part of me wasn't sure I liked all the hoopla. But I decided to go along with it and placed my index finger up against my temple and began tapping it. My father smiled.

"Can you do other things?" he asked excitedly. "Can you do bigger numbers?"

"I'll try," I told him.

He slowly wrote out a two-digit number beneath a three-digit one, multiplied them together and, after a bit of scribbling, wrote the answer down on another sheet of paper, not letting me see it. Not that I even thought about looking. When he pushed the page toward me, I instantly barked out the answer. My father just grinned, tousled my hair, and shouted: "Loveda, I want to show you something!"

Picking up his adding machine, pencil, and a piece of paper, my father motioned for me to follow him into the kitchen. My mother was standing by the sink, drying plates. She turned to find us sitting at the kitchen table, my father busily writing down more numbers.

"Jerry here has a pretty neat trick he can do," he said, not bothering to look up. "Watch."

He motions for me to do my stunt. This time he doesn't even wait for me to spout out my answer before he begins entering the numbers into his adding machine, which I've begun to think sounds like a tractor.

Long before he's finished, I pick up his pencil and write down a four-digit number at the bottom of the page. A moment later, my father is staring at the same number on the piece of paper draping out from his machine.

"I just don't know how he does it," he said, shaking his head.

My mother looked at me, trying to appear unfazed, but I could tell she was pleased. "Well," she said to my father. "We're both pretty good with numbers. I guess he will be, too."

I wondered if she was going to try to hug me but quickly realized there wasn't a chance of that. They both stared at me, smiling contentedly. Neither said a word. A moment later, I felt myself grow tired of the spotlight. I'd begun to feel like a circus freak. I walked back into the dining room, sat in my father's chair, and tried not to think about addition or multiplication. Our parakeet whistled a strange out-of-tune melody that I convinced myself was meant solely for me. Listening to the staccato bursts of sound, I drifted off, far away, far from the numbers, out into space.

ELK HORN, WISCONSIN
MARCH 1955

On the moon, the part of the moon that refuses to ever face Earth, exists a deep, obscure crater named after my grandfather. He was a world-renowned astronomer, best remembered for calculating the temperature of the sun. My father was also a famous astronomer, the kind who has an asteroid named after him. Given all the time that these two men spent peering into telescopes, staring into the heavens, it's appropriate that my first memory involves stars. Hundreds of them. Brilliant cadmium white flecks, pinpricks of light spinning and dancing in front of my eyes. So beautiful, really.

There's another good but strange reason why my first memory involved stars. It was due to one of my sisters accidentally dropping me on my head. It happened several months after my birth in Elk Horn, Wisconsin, where my father was heading up the observatory for the University of Chicago. Because my mother often worked through the night with my father at the observatory, she tried to catch a few hours of sleep during the afternoon. That was why my sister was rocking me in our family's new cradle on that hot afternoon—only it rocked much more vigorously than our previous one, swinging back and forth in huge, exaggerated arcs with only the slightest touch. Before long, the cradle flipped upside down, causing me to drop headfirst to the wood floor.

Terrified over what she'd done, she darted outside into the backyard. Then everything went black and I saw images that resembled stars flashing inside my head. I can still see myself lying there, staring up at the ceiling. The visuals resembled the Milky Way, expansive and shimmering.

Not long after I met him, I realized that Jerry was a stargazer, too. He had the ability to look up into the night sky and discern the shapes of animals—cartoon characters mostly—in the flickering heavens above. When he gazed up at the constellation Cassiopeia, he somehow visualized the image of Wonder Dog. Somewhere within the three bright stars Vega, Altair, and Deneb, he claimed to spy Felix the Cat. That was one of the sexiest things Jerry ever did for me—telling me how he spied all those goofy shapes in the heavens above. That sort of thing would have been absolute heresy in my family of no-nonsense, left-brained scientists.

Without question, we were a strange family. My parents reminded me of a cross between two clueless lab coat–clad scientists out of a *Far Side* cartoon and the brilliant Madame Curie and her husband, Pierre. None of us Meinels particularly fit in very well with the outside world. Yet in a family full of freaks, I definitely had my own tent at the carnival. For as long as I can remember, we always kept our distance from our neighbors. We moved a lot, hopping from one house to the next, each more remote than the previous one. By the time I became a toddler, my erratic behavior had earned me the nickname "circus monster." One minute I could be calm and tranquil, and the next, I'd explode into a seething dervish of unhinged chaos, much like Taz, the lovable, yet violently reactive Tasmanian devil in the Warner Brothers cartoons.

With a built-in home entertainment system like me in the family, it's no surprise that one of my six sibling's favorite hobbies was to call me names, then watch me emerge from my placid cocoon and fly into a psychotic rage. It didn't take much to send me off. The neighborhood kids would come over to watch, often joining the fun. They'd pick up a chair to play lion tamer with me, trying to goad me into one of my explosive spasms that would send me running around the room shrieking. My older sister Carolyn was the only sibling who didn't participate in my torture sessions. She didn't always come to my rescue, but the others seemed to understand that Carolyn didn't approve of the torment they inflicted upon me. All it took was a few seconds of her withering stare to diffuse the situation.

Then again, my siblings were often even more brutal to each other—pummeling one another with their fists and other objects. In one pitched battle, Elaine and Wally went after each other with baseball bats. My siblings were equally ruthless when it came to playing board games like Risk, where the only way you can win is through betrayal, a skill I never could master despite being surrounded by those to whom it came so easily. Family game nights would reduce me to a sobbing, gasping wreck.

When I was two, we moved to Scottsdale, where my father was hired as a professor at the University of Arizona's Kitt Peak National Observatory. Not long afterward, my weary mother began locking herself in the bathroom in a desperate attempt for a respite from me. It never worked. I quickly learned how to jimmy open any bathroom or bedroom door. I used to follow her around the house seeking attention like a puppy. She would look at me for a brief moment, scoot me out into the backyard, and instruct me to go entertain myself. Then she'd lock me out of the house. It took me years to figure out how to open the complicated lock on that sliding glass door.

When I was three, my father was sitting in a chair near the fireplace. Overjoyed to have him all to myself, I ran across the room, jumped in his lap, and kissed him. He slapped me, then shoved me away. I tried to convince myself that I must have bitten him. The alternative was too tough to contemplate. But now I think I know the real reason—my father had sensory issues of his own. He struck me and pushed me away out of panic, not maliciousness. He was terrified of being hugged, although my siblings could, on rare occasions, sneak one in if they approached him slowly, cautiously, almost the way one would a skittish rabbit or a nervous cat. Unfortunately, I was much too impulsive for those sorts of niceties. As a result of that rebuff, I grew so angry at my parents that inside my head I never allowed myself to use the term mom or dad. Instead, I always referred to them as Marjorie and Dr. Meinel.

One afternoon while my father was searching for a site on which to locate the University of Arizona's new observatory, he caught a spotted black skunk up on Kitt Peak. He took the animal back to our house as a gift for us kids and locked him up in a cage in the corner of the backyard. And that's when I finally got my first real friend—a skunk. After that, whenever my mom locked me out of the house, I'd sit beside his little wire cage and lose myself, staring into his dark eyes that resembled two black oil-drenched marbles. I never realized that he could have sprayed me with his stench.

It was during one of those backyard exiles that I first discovered the transformative powers of sound. My instrument of choice was a wooden picnic table sitting in the middle of our property near the massive vegetable garden where my mother grew most of our food. One afternoon, I grew so bored sitting outside by myself that I happened to press my ear down against the splintered planks of the table. What I heard amazed me—all sorts of low, guttural rumblings that seemed to be coming up through the wood. The more I moved my head, the more the tones would change in pitch. Before long, I began whiling away the hot afternoons listening to the picnic table, looking at the world sideways, losing myself in those fascinating moans that I later learned—after one of Marjorie's scientific lectures—were caused by air compression changes that made my eardrum bend, much in the same way that listening to a seashell does.

The yard behind our home eventually became my domain. My mother didn't need to lock the door anymore because I was no longer interested in venturing inside. I'd finally discovered a haven, safe from my siblings—or at least it was most of the time. I can still remember that afternoon, when my brother Wally shattered my calm. He was heading off to do battle with a group of kids in a nearby housing development, and I desperately wanted to accompany him. But he refused, due to the fact that I was such a pathetic fighter and he knew my presence would distract him when the blows and dirt clods began flying. When I refused to take no for an answer, he began to fight with me.

A few minutes into it, I glanced over the ranch-style fence on the edge of our property. Four neighborhood toughs, all in their teens, were leaning up against the wooden rails, watching my beating. As usual, my face was dirty and streaked with tears. I'd been whipped up into one of my typical rages, but in between my sobbing gasps, I found myself studying their curious faces. Tormenting a younger sibling is, of course, a universal rite of passage for both parties. But something about their expressions told me they'd clearly never seen anything quite like this. Something told me they felt embarrassed.

"Knock it off, Wally," the largest boy shouted. "Leave your sister alone." He paused, then leaned over the fence as if he were going to climb into the front yard. "You understand what I'm saying ... *play nice!*"

I turned to watch what sort of effect the words would have on my brother. At the time, Wally was circling his prey, preparing to deliver his usual deathblow. But suddenly he was frozen dead in his tracks, staring sheepishly at the ground and mumbling something I couldn't quite hear. A moment later, he fled inside the house and I was left wondering if everyone's life felt quite as hopeless as mine.

Around the age of three, I discovered the wonder of visual arts, thanks to an enormous oil painting hanging on our living room wall, up above the sofa. For much of my childhood, I could often be found with my face pressed up against it, lost in a universe created by a painter who signed his name as Cryl E. Baker. This simple landscape, depicting a single, enormous mountain rising up out of a gentle grassland, spoke to me in a language that I instantly understood, a language that went way beyond words. Scraggly evergreens sprouted from the craggy sides of the rocky peak. The sky wasn't blue, but glowed a murky shade of green. All around our home in Scottsdale, we were surrounded by mountains, but none remotely resembled the one depicted on our wall. The true genius of the painting, the part that drew me into it like a fleck of iron to a magnet, was this nearly microscopic horse and rider depicted in the foreground, just off to the right. How could this Cryl E. Baker perform such magic on a piece of canvas that measured five feet by three feet?

At first glance, the painting seemed intent on drawing my eye to the massive peak dominating the canvas. Yet my eyes always rested upon that solitary rider as he slowly made his way toward the peak looming in the distance. It was midday in the painting, and he wore a strange-looking hat and a muted red coat, a wardrobe choice that struck me as truly amazing. Why would a painter need to clad such a diminutive subject in a brilliantly colored cloak?

For hours at a time I'd stare into this landscape the way much of my family would watch television. I'd carefully, painstakingly inspect each individual brushstroke, thrilled by the genius and craftsmanship of how the paint rose up off the canvas. Every atom, every burst of color seemed enigmatically alive. I didn't feel myself pulled inside the picture. Rather, this painting seemed to somehow reach deep into my brain, gently asking me to experience exactly what it felt like to be that lone rider, to be so tiny, yet so omnipresent as I moved toward something so much larger than myself.

I admired my older siblings, even though they never wanted anything to do with me. They were all talented artists, and I spent much of my time literally trying to copy everything they did. Elaine would fashion entire villages out of clay and populate them with countless handmade people. But of all my brothers and sisters, Carolyn was the one true shining light. She tolerated me in a way that sometimes made me feel as though she actually enjoyed my company. We planted gardens together. She taught me how to

soak the ground before plowing it. We raised chickens and pheas-
ants. Sometimes, when she'd return home from school in the afternoons, we'd take our chickens walking around the block. Just the
two us and our herd of poultry. Sometimes, my father would take
his axe out from the garage and lop off one of our roosters' heads.
That sort of thing never bothered Carolyn.

One afternoon, when I was four, my mother loaded me and
my younger brother, David, into our Plymouth station wagon and
pointed it in the direction of Townsend Junior High School, where
Carolyn attended eighth grade.

"Carolyn fell asleep in class," my mother mumbled without
a hint of emotion. It took us fifteen minutes to make the drive
across town to the school.

Moments after we pulled up to the school entrance, two men
emerged through the heavy swinging front doors. They were carrying Carolyn's limp body. One clutched her ankles. The other
held her arms. Carolyn sagged in the middle like a bag of chicken
feed, and they loaded her into the back of the station wagon, then
slammed the tailgate shut. Nobody said much of anything. At least
nothing I could understand. My mother turned on the radio and
drove. I sat on my knees, pressing my stomach against the backseat,
staring down at Carolyn, gently touching her wispy, blond hair with
my fingertips. I couldn't figure out why she wouldn't open her eyes.

We dropped her off at the hospital. I watched my mother disappear inside for a few minutes, then suddenly reappear. On the
drive back home, my mother would say nothing about our sister.
Carolyn spent most of the next year sealed off from the world
in a coma. I missed her horribly. The only member of my family
who had ever treated me with any kindness had gone away and
I couldn't understand why. None of us kids could. Whenever
we asked Marjorie and Dr. Meinel what had happened, we received various answers. There were two repeated causes for her
deep sleep. She had been bitten by a tsetse fly, causing Carolyn
to contract encephalitis. The other excuse centered upon the idea

that she'd gone so stark raving mad that the circuitry in her brain had overloaded, then permanently gone on the fritz. After a few months, we all began to accept the latter hypothesis.

Before long, Carolyn's coma marked the beginning of what became a wildly popular story line in our family—the insanity offense. My father possessed a deep, dark fear that running through the bloodline of our family was an insanity gene. If one of us kids did anything out of line, acted peculiar, or exhibited any sort of behavior that proved offensive to Marjorie and Dr. Meinel, we were declared insane, schizophrenic, or hallucinatory. I quickly grew to fear being called crazy. It meant just one thing—deep, perpetual sleep.

More than anything, I wanted Carolyn to wake up and come back home. I used to beg Marjorie to drive me to the hospital to see her. One morning, we drove to the hospital and I stood in the lobby, staring at the elevator doors, waiting for them to slide open, waiting for my sister to appear. When those doors finally opened, I couldn't believe what I saw. Carolyn was awake, but just barely. Her body sat limp and tiny in a wheelchair, like a wilted plant. Those beautiful blue eyes of hers were glazed and rolled up in her head, staring listlessly at the ceiling. In the months that had passed since she'd drifted away, her lungs had atrophied and filled with fluid. I could hear her raspy, labored breathing.

When she finally arrived home from the hospital, she wasn't the same Carolyn. She began drawing and painting for the first time in her life, and it took her another year before she fully returned to us. My mother would stuff her full of amphetamines, trying to keep her awake, but she'd always just drift off. I think I was jealous. I wanted to follow her to wherever she kept escaping, to whatever place kept drawing her back.

We shared a bedroom together after her coma. "I missed you," I'd tell her. "Where did you go? Tell me where you went."

She couldn't remember much, insisting that her only souvenir from the whole odyssey was a faint memory of a recurring dream. In it, she was a dog, walking into a beautifully lush forest, sponge-like soil beneath her feet, dark green fir trees towering paternally overhead. All at once, the forest began to transform itself into a barren, parched field. At the same time, she watched herself morph into a wolf and before long she was standing in the middle of a World War II battlefield, the air filled with acrid smoke, white-hot shards of metal flying through the air. She couldn't escape. There was nowhere to run or hide.

What Carolyn must have endured during her strange journey I couldn't understand—but I identified with her. I felt different, too. The problem was, I just couldn't put my finger on how. Even more confusing, I didn't have a coma to blame for it.

By then, I avoided my siblings at all cost, choosing instead to spend my time with our dalmation, Lady, and our cat, Tom. If I wasn't hiding out in the backyard, I'd lie down on the living room floor on top of an old parachute, petting them for hours, whispering nice things into their tiny ears, things I thought they wanted to hear, things I always wanted people to say to me. I was off the family radar. I'd disappeared. Often, I'd imagine myself on a horse, riding high into the local mountains somewhere, far away from my peculiar family.

Sometimes I'd wander over to our ancient Baldwin baby grand piano that had once belonged to my father's mother and touch the keys. Even though it was horribly out of tune because my father hadn't touched it since returning from the war, the sounds it created were more wondrous than anything I'd ever experienced. The overtones and beat rates were hypnotic, alluring.

We were a religious family, strict Lutherans who attended church every Sunday. Church was the one place where I never found it difficult to sit still. Something about the Gregorian chants worked like a sonic tranquilizer on my chaotic mind. The organ music mesmerized me. By an early age, I'd managed to memorize nearly fifteen minutes' worth of the chants. Whenever I found myself in need of peace and calm, I'd mouth these ancient Latin melodic hymns, desperately praying that the serenity I'd felt in church would wash over me like the buckets of water my brothers would toss on me.

Despite the lack of communication in our family, I was fascinated by language and interpreted everything I heard literally. This trait became awkwardly apparent one Saturday afternoon as my parents and siblings were gathered around our massive TV set, staring at a discus thrower on *ABC's Wide World of Sports*. Suddenly, the announcer screamed: "He just broke the record! He shattered the record!" Everyone in my family began cheering and clapping. I can do that, I thought to myself, and quickly wandered to the back of the living room and began pulling out Marjorie's collection of 78s and 33s. Stacking as many records as I could in my younger brother David's outstretched arms, we walked out the front door and sat down in the middle of the lawn, carefully pulling them out from their paper sleeves. Everyone was too engrossed in the flickering black-and-white TV screen to notice us. I'm not sure how many of her records we demolished on our concrete driveway that afternoon, but every time they'd splinter into pieces on the concrete driveway, I'd cheer: "I just broke the record! I just broke the record!"

By first grade, I'd begun to realize that I'd become my family's most annoying problem. No one knew what to do with me. I'd sit in class at my little desk and feel a part of me lifting out of my body, floating off into outer space, out among the stars. This was why I often never replied when my teacher asked me a question, which led to her diagnosis that I must be deaf. I was repeatedly sent to the nurse's office, where I'd have headphones clamped over my ears and a palate of tones pumped into my head. I was anything but deaf. In reality, I possessed the hearing of a wild animal and those tones, especially the high ones, felt like someone was driving an ice pick through my head. Eventually, I was sent to a hearing specialist for more tests. He sat me down on his examination table and patiently explained what each of the tests would entail. Then he walked my mother to the back of the room and quietly whispered, "Do you think she'd like a sucker when we're done with the tests?"

"I'd love a sucker!" I exclaimed happily.

They both looked over at me incredulously, then at each other. The doctor shrugged. "I don't really think she needs a hearing test," he announced.

That was the last time anyone suggested that my ears might be the cause of my peculiar behavior. After that, the search for excuses ended. I was just a weird kid, a hopeless misfit. End of story.

CHAPTER THREE

 Late morning, just before lunch. A teacher armed with a shiny metal whistle directed twenty-six second graders down a clean linoleum-lined hallway and out onto the playground for recess, which was definitely not my best subject. I wandered past the jungle gyms and swing sets, out onto the expanse of hard-packed dirt where we played team sports.

Mary wouldn't have fared very well on our playground. It hurts me to think about what would have happened if she'd somehow been magically transported there. I miraculously possessed just enough diplomatic skills to steer clear of many of the social land mines that would have ripped apart someone like her. When I think about how badly she would have been teased and picked on, it makes tears well up in my eyes. I ask myself sometimes, What would I have done for her? I'd like to think I would have protected her, but I was so full of confusion and self-hate back then that there's really no telling how I would have reacted. And that saddens me.

On that particular spring morning out behind the Wingamhauppaugue Elementary School, all the other boys were busy choosing sides for baseball, one of my favorite sports. I tried not to let myself wonder whether I'd get picked for a team. The guys never totally ignored me. They just usually stuck me out into very distant deep right field or another position where I could do the least amount of damage.

I was standing there studying a clump of dirt, waiting to see what team got stuck with me, when I heard the sound of sneakers approaching from behind.

"Here he is," explained a voice I'd never heard before. "Here's the kid I was telling you about."

I spun around in time to see four older kids approaching—three boys and a girl. I knew what was about to happen and without thinking I immediately began staring bashfully down at my feet. My heart beat crazily and I felt myself wondering how one could both love and hate something so much. A moment later, they surrounded me.

"Hey, Newport, do your trick for Johnny, here," one of them commanded. "Show him your number thing. Do some big numbers."

A jolt of electricity pulsed through my body. I suddenly felt powerful, wanted, and accepted and tried to convince myself that I actually believed everything my head was trying to tell me. I took a deep breath.

"You have to give me the numbers," I reminded him.

"Oh, yeah," he says. "That's right."

I stood there, waiting forever for him to come up with some random numbers, trying to ignore the feeling rising up inside me.

"Okay, here's one," he said. "What's three hundred twenty-five times one thousand and thirteen?"

I tried to smile at my inquisitors, but I doubt that the expression on my face resembled anything close to a smile. All the while, the numbers crawled their way deep inside my head and went about their business, doing just what they were supposed to do.

Back then, I envisioned the process as something similar to how my stomach always knew how to digest food after I swallowed it. It all happened so far off in the background that I didn't bother paying attention to it. And just as my stomach understood what it needed to do, so did my brain. That was why I never uttered any of the numbers that were thrown at me. That was what made me different from others who tried to do calculations inside their heads. It was the vocalization that slowed people down.

A few brief seconds later, I spouted out the answer. "It's 329,225," I told them. All three looked amazed, although I wondered how they truly knew my answer was correct. I'd already become such a mythic playground oddity that nobody even questioned the accuracy of my answers anymore. Not that the questions I was asked were all that difficult. It certainly didn't take much to impress the elementary school crowd. Rarely did I get anything larger than a five-digit number tossed at me.

A hand slapped me on the back. "You ever seen anything like that?" the boy said to his companions. "Newport is a walking adding machine. Isn't that crazy? Isn't that just the craziest thing you ever saw?"

His companions stared at me like one would an animal in the zoo and shook their heads in disbelief; then they walked away, and I stood there watching their backs, listening to their whispers.

"Yeah, I heard about him," a voice said. "But I didn't think it was real.... How's he do that?"

"Don't ask me," his pal whispered. "But he's kind of a nut job." He placed his index finger up next to his temple, then whirred it around in a circle, the universal sign for crazy.

Then they were gone. The floodwaters of attention suddenly dried up and I was left standing there alone—Jerry Newport, the fascinating genius, had been transformed back into Jerry Newport, the lonely freak. One moment I was popular, the next a pariah. One moment I would be basking in all the attention a kid could ever want, the next nobody would talk to me. Why couldn't

I have been good at something useful? Why couldn't I be a base-ball savant? Several decades passed before I realized that it was okay to be a geek, just as long as you don't hate yourself for it the way I did.

It didn't take long for word of my peculiar skill to leak out. Within a couple weeks of my father's having me perform for my mother, everyone in the community seemed to be whispering about it, which wasn't entirely surprising. My parents always treated my brothers and me like little trophies, objects they could show off to make them feel good. My mother especially lived for this sort of recognition. She wanted to push the envelope and see how far I could go with my gift for numbers. My uncanny ability to crunch numbers made her feel better about herself. When the other moth-ers would compliment her for my ability, she got to feign mod-esty, which was something she loved to do. My parents even toyed with the possibility of having me appear on Ted Mack's *Origi-nal Amateur Hour*, a national broadcast TV talent show taped in Manhattan. My father eventually nixed the idea. He sensed my discomfort over becoming a sideshow freak on television, which was something he could relate to. He didn't have time for show-offs. Deep down, I think he truly wanted me to put my brain in deep freeze until the rest of the world could catch up with me. Even back then, I sensed that this said more about how he viewed himself than what he thought of me.

What frustrated and saddened me most was the feeling that I was doing nothing with my gift. If I'd been a prodigy baseball player, I never would have been stuck playing in a league where I could run, throw, and hit circles around the other players. Surely my talent would have been noticed and I would have been moved up to a league with better players, older players. Why couldn't my parents do that with me academically, helping me make the most of my gifts, instead of allowing me to spend most of my school career sitting around and waiting for the other kids to catch up?

As time went by, I became yet another one of those math whizzes who dreaded attending math class. While all my classmates were struggling to learn their multiplication tables, I was chomping on my no. 2 pencil to sink my teeth into geometry, algebra, trigonometry, and calculus. I'd sit at my desk, wondering why nobody was paying attention to me. Am I really that much of a freak? One day, just before the end of second grade, my mother had an idea. She was teaching eighth-grade math at the time and thought it might be interesting to have me take the screening test used for kids trying to get into private schools. I breezed through it and easily managed to score as high as any of the students in her class.

"That's very good, Jerry," she told me after learning about my results. And that was that. Nothing more was said about the issue.

Despite his lack of patience and occasional flashes of temper, my dad was sensitive to my frustrations and feelings of intellectual alienation. Roughly six months after the discovery of my savant powers, he began trying to get me interested in sports statistics. He knew intuitively that it would provide me with an outlet to use my gift in a way my friends could relate to. Each evening, I'd comb through the sports pages of *Newsday,* devouring every article, plucking out any numerical stat I could unearth. I never purposely tried to memorize the data, but when it came to numbers I soaked them up. Once they lodged inside my head, they stayed. Before long, I became a walking encyclopedia of sports trivia, particularly adept in the realm of track and field. I could recite the numerical details behind each world record, in every event. The sensation of having all that data lodged inside my head gave me an indescribable feeling of control. For the first time in my life, I could impose some sense of order on a universe that often felt entirely chaotic.

And there was nothing I craved more than order and control. I remember once holding an acorn in my hand, measuring it solely by using my mind, then spending the next few hours calculating exactly how many similarly sized acorns it would take to fill up the top drawer of my bedside table. I loved studying the symmetry of the leaves, following the network of veinlike ridges that forked and multiplied across their surfaces in every imaginable direction. In the afternoons when school let out, I went to the garage and turned my bicycle upside down on the concrete floor. I'd crank the pedals with my hands and watch the back wheel spin itself into a blur in front of my face. In a corner of the garage sat my mother's washing machine. The moment I'd hear it whirring into its spin cycle, I'd run over, yank open the lid, and try to guess what color would catch my eye first. White socks? A red T-shirt? A pair of blue jeans? My father's red-checkered boxer shorts? Sometimes the fluttery feeling of anticipation inside my stomach just before some article of clothing came into view was almost unbearable. The possibility of controlling an object in motion was gloriously addictive. I craved it in a way I couldn't explain.

Everyone's life can be broken down into chapters. For me, a new chapter started one afternoon toward the end of third grade when a group of neighborhood kids, along with my brothers, discovered my upside-down bicycle in the garage and wheeled it out into the driveway. Up until that point, my bicycle had always served as a powerful symbol in my life. All the other kids knew how to ride, but not me. Years before, I learned to dread that moment when we'd all be goofing around in somebody's yard and everyone began hopping on their bikes. It meant that whatever time I had with those few kids who would tolerate me was now officially over. They would ride off down the street, leaving me alone for the rest of the day.

But on that particular afternoon, things took a different twist. "It's time you learned how to ride this thing, Newport," said Alfred, a hell-raising Eddie Haskell sort who lived a few blocks away. "Get on."

I stared at him, waiting for him to come to his senses. After all, everyone knew I possessed the coordination of a drunken elephant. The notion of my attempting to balance my body on those two skinny tires seemed theoretically impossible. Alfred, however, wasn't in the mood for excuses. Neither were his buddies. So I did as I was told and climbed onto the seat. Five pairs of hands (fifty fingers) clutched the frame of my bike.

"Okay, Newport, we're going to walk with you and you're going to go faster and faster," explained Alfred, as he pushed and pulled my legs up and down on the pedals. "When we get going fast enough, we're going to let go and you're going to keep going all by yourself."

For once, I didn't have time to consult my brain. Everything was unfolding far too quickly. I was petrified. But the farther we journeyed down Oak Tree Lane, the more I began to enjoy the rhythm of my legs pushing the pedals. Then, before I realized it, the hands clutching my bike let go and I continued sailing down the street, free as a bird, perfectly balanced. I could hear cheering behind me. I never wanted to stop moving, but at the end of the block I pushed on the brakes and turned the bike around. My heart nearly beat itself out of my chest. Sir Edmund Hillary must have felt like this that day he stood on top of Mount Everest. Nothing was ever the same again.

Once I learned how to ride a bike, my universe immediately changed. Before long I got a paper route just like my brother Jim and pedaled around the neighborhood, delivering copies of *Newsday* every day after school. It taught me some precious lessons about life.

Harassment comes with the job when you're a paperboy. My first hurdle was the neighborhood canines who could sense my basic physical insecurity, often charging my bike along the route. Then, of course, there were the kids who would gang up on me as I wheeled past their houses with my bag full of papers slung off my back. I became the perfect moving target for rocks and mud balls. But something snapped the day Vinny, a former friend who'd been forced to repeat fourth grade, tried running me off the road on his bike. A part of me decided that it was time to fight back.

"You're a dead duck, Newport," he shouted, as he rode beside me, trying to kick me over and using his front wheel as a battering ram to break out my spokes. My mother had always told me to avoid incidents like this—just to ignore the bullies and go about my business. But something told me that approach was only going to make matters worse. So I slammed on my brakes and came to a quick stop. Surprised, Vinny slowed down, then came to a sloppy stop and glared at me.

"What's your problem?" I shouted.

"I . . . I don't like you, Newport," he said.

"I don't really like you either, right now," I stammered, a rage building up inside of me.

"I don't care," he said, walking toward me. "Gimme your papers."

I snapped. If I let him take my papers, that was it. I may as well give up my *Newsday* route because from that day forward I'd be a sitting duck for every kid who wanted to pick on somebody. I clutched my bag against my side, ran awkwardly straight at Vinny, and kicked him in the shin. He looked stunned. Then I pushed over his bike.

"I'm really sorry you got held back, Vinny," I screamed. "But that's not my problem. . . . Nobody's taking my newspapers."

"Shut up, Newport," he said, picking up his bike, inspecting his chipped-up paint job. "You—you scratched my bike."

But by then I'd climbed back on my bike and had begun pedaling down the street. A fragile, uneasy peace had been reached. No use in hanging around. I wiped the tears out of my eyes, reached into my bag, and grabbed a newspaper, then heaved it like a grenade up onto a nearby lawn. Tears were streaming down my face, but I didn't feel sad.

⌇

When it came to my own feelings, I was a sensitive kid. Whatever emotion—no matter how subtle—washed through my head or heart, I felt it with bewildering clarity. Yet I was often clueless about what other people were feeling. My lack of empathy wasn't intentional. It just took longer for data, such as someone else's emotions, to worm its way into my brain. When it did, when it finally worked its way inside the part of me that allowed me to experience empathy, I felt awful. Once, when my father and I were out running an errand in town, we came upon several ambulances and a group of policemen. A young boy, the brother of a kid I attended elementary school with, had just been hit by a car and killed. I stood there watching the boy's father go into hysterics over the death of his boy. He sobbed and gasped. One of the police officers had to hold him up to keep him from collapsing on the sidewalk. The next morning, before school started, I stood under a stairwell with some friends and launched into what I thought was a hilarious imitation of the grief-stricken father.

"So, who died?" I was asked.

"Linda Morton's little brother," I replied, miffed that my routine had been interrupted. "I think his name was Billy."

A look of sadness swept across the faces of my friends. "I know him," Johnny Aichroth whispered. "Uh, I knew him. . . . He was a great little kid."

Nobody said another word. One by one, they all walked away. In a flash, I felt awful. Up until that moment, I'd never connected all the dots. I never considered that Billy Morton had been a real person. It never occurred to me that the reason his father was so upset was because his son had just been killed. I truly believed that I was just re-creating a scene, almost like a TV set, letting my friends experience what I'd seen the previous afternoon. For the next few days, I felt sick to my stomach over what I'd done. I wanted to apologize, but I never did. I didn't know what to say or who to say it to.

For me, feeling other people's pain, being cognizant of other people's emotions has been a learned skill. I literally did not feel pain. Once, while swinging from a rope tied to the limb of a maple tree in our backyard, I fell and split the back of my head open on the metal lid of the septic tank. I got up and started climbing back up into the tree when I noticed Jim appeared on the verge of passing out. Something about the expression on his face made me place my hand on the back of my head, which was soaked with blood. It finally dawned on me what had happened. I screamed. A half hour later I was stretched out on a gurney at a local hospital, having my head stitched up.

"I just don't understand it," my mother said to a nurse as the doctor wrapped a white gauze bandage around my head. "He just doesn't feel pain when he's supposed to." The doctor didn't seem to have a clue about what she was talking about. He just stood there nodding as my mother talked; then he patted me on the shoulder and disappeared down the hallway to his next patient.

Often in class, while the rest of the kids were struggling to finish a reading assignment that I'd breezed through long ago, I'd sit there glaring at everyone, waiting for them to finish. And that's when I'd begin yanking off any and all scabs that happened to be on my elbows or arms, then pop them into my mouth. It was a nervous habit, something I was powerless to control. Sometimes the freshly opened wounds would begin to bleed, but I never felt anything. It was as if I were watching the whole thing on a movie screen, like it was happening to someone else.

Which isn't to say that somewhere deep inside of me, in that quiet place far removed from that part of me that crunched numbers and absorbed statistical data, I didn't yearn to feel what others felt, in real time. In that daydream world located smack dab in the middle of my head, I helped people, not hurt them. I used to have dreams back then, recurring action-adventure shows in my head, where I played the role of a giant whale that did nothing but good for others. I rescued smaller fish by using my enormous head as a battering ram against the trawlers that would hunt them. Sometimes I'd save the occasional human from drowning and dismemberment by hungry sharks, by carrying him back to shore on my back.

A part of me was nothing more than an exposed, raw nerve, especially when an insult or slight was thrown my way. When that happened, the hurt washed over me like a tidal wave. It engulfed me, threatening to pull me under and keep me there forever.

Sometimes I'd suffer in silence. Other times, I'd explode in consuming rages. By the time I reached junior high, I'd cemented my reputation as someone with a hair-trigger temper that could be set off for no apparent reason. Sometimes I'd react with physical violence. For example, whenever I'd miss a note on my trombone, I'd slam the slide down onto the floor, which quickly bent it at a ridiculous angle.

Other times, I'd erupt with strings of obscenities. One evening at Boy Scout camp, a few of my buddies were tormenting the fifteen-year-old counselor.

"Hey, Newport, cuss him out," one of them said.

I looked at the counselor for a moment and quickly felt the familiar rage building up inside of me. A moment later, curse words were erupting out of me like shrapnel from a grenade. Once started, I couldn't stop myself. I felt powerless. After a few moments, my friends grew bored of the show and wandered back to their cabin. But the counselor just stood there, staring at me wide-eyed as I continued spewing forth my rage-filled lexicon.

"Why would you say that?" he asked, shaking his head in bewilderment.

Drained of my venom, I grew quiet. I couldn't move. Suddenly, I started to cry. Why had I just done that? Why had I just attacked a complete stranger?

Yet it was the quiet rages that hurt me most, the stints of self-loathing that stung me deeper than any verbal or physical tantrum. Like that Saturday afternoon my brothers and I drove out to the local speedway in John's new Austin to watch the stock car races.

My all-time favorite driver was the spunky Japanese racer George Tet, who was forever going head-to-head against all the other redneck racers on the circuit. Even then, I loved the underdog. I could relate. At a break in the racing, I ventured up to the restroom to empty my Coca-Cola-filled bladder. Standing there at the urinal, I heard snickering and muffled laughter. I had a hunch why. When it came to personal plumbing, I wasn't the most well endowed of kids. Nevertheless, I couldn't believe that people could be so cruel and sadistic. I turned to see a couple of kids I knew standing there, staring at my private parts, smirking. Fighting the urge to break into tears, I stumbled out of the restroom, into the exhaust smoke and sunshine.

"Where you going, Jerry?" shouted one of my tormentors.

I didn't reply. I couldn't. I yearned to climb over the racetrack fence and hurl myself in front of the cars, but I was too afraid of heights to pull it off. Instead, I walked through the dirt, past the concession stand, hoping to find a place under the bleachers where I could hide, where I could feel inferior and ashamed all by myself.

TUCSON, ARIZONA
APRIL 1964

A ghost. That was what I'd become by the time elementary school got ahold of me. I smelled pretty bad, too. My mother had a million other things to do besides monitoring my hygiene. My hands and fingernails often looked as though I moonlighted as a mechanic. And my mother would slather my defiant cowlick, which her home haircuts couldn't control, with an industrial-strength Vaseline-like substance that resembled automotive grease. My wardrobe usually consisted of oversized hand-me-downs from older sisters. Teachers were alarmed. Classmates either steered clear of me or teased me mercilessly.

What would Jerry have done if he'd seen me back then? That's what I sometimes ask myself. Sure, I needed a bath. But what I needed even more was a friend. I can't help thinking that Jerry would have been that friend. I tell myself that if the two of us had somehow come in contact with each other, we would have been drawn together like two magnets. I want to believe that's true because I want that filthy, lonely little girl who lives deep inside my head to have someone like Jerry, to know someone who will convince her that she's not the circus freak everyone wanted her to believe she was.

Back then, back in elementary school, I was a big kid with a body that walked that fine line between overweight and obese. Kids called me names like "wide load" and "Meinel-ephant." By fourth grade, I still enjoyed pretending to be an infant and thought nothing of crawling around on the carpeted floor like a helpless, clueless toddler. The sensation of the carpet fibers rubbing against my body felt soft, comforting. We had a stable behind our house, and I could often be found there wandering around in the yard on all fours, pretending to be a horse.

In fifth grade, my teacher, Mrs. Young, a former soybean farmer who moved to Arizona to escape the merciless winters of Iowa, saw something in me that nobody else did. My voracious curiosity intrigued her. She began to instruct me on how to wash beneath my fingernails and why I shouldn't sit at my desk with my legs spread apart. One day, she knocked on the front door of our house and attempted to speak with my mother about her strange, dirty daughter who possessed an innate knack for drawing. Mrs. Young particularly liked the horses I used to sketch in class and once even went to the trouble of showing them to a professor at the University of Arizona's art department, who stopped by my class one day, stood by my desk, and told me what a good artist I was.

"Keep on drawing and maybe you'll see your pictures hanging in a museum one day," I recall her whispering to me. Because I didn't have much experience with compliments, I had no idea what to make of her kind words. So I turned away from her and continued staring out the window, looking for pictures in the clouds.

My parents weren't impressed with my skill. Nor were they surprised by it. They would have been surprised if I hadn't been an amazing artist. The only pictures drawn by any of us kids that they saw fit to display on the walls of our house were the portraits Carolyn had painted of her pheasant, created after she emerged from her coma.

Mrs. Young's conversation with my mother lasted only a couple of minutes. Marjorie apparently figured that if my teacher had nothing better to do than to fritter away a nice afternoon with her uncontrollable daughter, she certainly wasn't going to stop her. I was crawling around on a bale of alfalfa in the tack room when Mrs. Young wandered into the stable looking for me.

"Why aren't you inside?" she asked. "It's cold out here."

"I like it out here," I replied. "I like it better than ... than being inside there." I motioned toward our house with my dirty hand, much like someone would point to a dead animal.

"Yes," she said, smiling. "I understand."

We walked out into the rock-strewn desert and she listened while I told her how at home I felt out among the ocotillo and barrel cactuses. As usual, I didn't wear any shoes. My feet were tough like leather. We walked through the foothills of the Catalina Mountains, and I pointed out where I had found giant sheets of mica and desert tortoises and how the century-old saguaros that towered over our heads weren't quite as threatening as they looked. I'd lean against them and show her how the old, brittle syringelike needles would crack off long before puncturing your skin.

The Hohokam Indians had lived out in this patch of desert for centuries, and I took her to the place where Carolyn and I had once discovered the remnants of some ancient foundations, along with countless pottery shards. I wondered how they managed to survive out here in this parched, inhospitable ovenlike land. I'd been attempting to survive in a different type of desert, too.

"Aren't you afraid of the rattlesnakes?" Mrs. Young asked.

I shook my head and told her how I sometimes killed them with rocks, then peeled their skins off and dried their skins in the sun by nailing them up on the wooden slats of our corral.

"I eat them," I told her proudly. "I boil up their carcasses and make rattlesnake stew. It tastes pretty much like chicken. It seems exotic."

"Yes," Mrs. Young said, nodding approvingly. "That's what I hear."

I'd never met a teacher like Mrs. Young. Deep down, I think she liked the way I blurted out whatever was percolating inside my head. Yet I couldn't understand why this woman wanted to reach out to me. Her caring words and reassuring facial expressions bounced off me. I was impervious to her compassion, oblivious to what she was trying to do for me. Today, I can't help thinking how different my life would have been if I had responded—even for an instant—and taken hold of the life ring she offered. The experience, no matter how fleeting, would have forever changed me. I would have tasted her kindness, enjoyed the flavor, and no doubt begun searching for others who could serve up the same dish.

What Mrs. Young saw in me was a raw glimmer of possibility that nobody else could, that not even I had ever glimpsed. When she asked that art professor to come to tell me how much promise I showed as an artist, she assumed she was doing me a favor, pumping me up, letting me know that there were things I could do that others couldn't. But she probably needn't have bothered. Besides my obliviousness, deep down I was an awful skeptic. Even at that relatively young age, I was already too stuffed full of self-doubt to listen to compliments. When it came to contemplating my skills as an artist, I'd already thrown in the towel and it was all Michelangelo's fault. Sure, I knew I could literally sketch circles around my classmates. But any sense of satisfaction or personal worth that it brought me changed the moment I discovered a book

on our living room coffee table that traced Michelangelo's development as an artist. I cracked it open but stopped a few pages later
in awestruck horror after glimpsing some pictures of sketches and
sculptures he'd created when he was my age. His ability to create
three-dimensionality, shadowing, and semiluminescence in whatever medium he worked boggled my mind. From that point on,
his intimidating specter hung over everything I ever created. In the
scope of real, lasting art, I reasoned that I was nothing but a crude
hack.

I felt a similar pang of loathing about my piano playing. In
fifth grade, I composed a dark ditty, "Misery River," that won an
honorable mention in a district-wide composition contest. When
the district superintendent learned that I'd never taken any lessons, he wrote my mother a letter urging her to find me a piano
teacher. This was right around the same time that my parents,
who worshiped baroque music, purchased a harpsichord for
the wife of our pastor at the Calvalry Lutheran Church. Before
I knew it, Mrs. Jorstaad had agreed to become my teacher and
I dutifully set out to hone my music skills with her. Then one
day I experienced another one of those bubble-bursting Michelangelo moments and any thoughts that I might possess a gift for
music evaporated. I convinced myself that I didn't really possess
the finesse to move my stubby fingers over a keyboard the way a
gifted pianist should. I also convinced myself that the reason I
sometimes missed notes was because I just didn't have the innate
ability to memorize where my fingers were supposed to land on
the keyboard. The final blow came when I admitted to myself
that I couldn't actually feel the rhythmic beats in the music. It
just didn't come naturally to me. I had to literally force myself
to *hear* the beats. From what I knew about classical music after
listening to those few albums I hadn't shattered, that sort of
shortcoming was blasphemy. It was the final straw that forced me
to stop dreaming about one day becoming a concert pianist. Of
course, it probably didn't help much that Marjorie warned me

not to become a child prodigy, insisting that they all end up going insane, burning out and, eventually, lapsing into hopeless mediocrity. In a way, I took her advice as a compliment. Although her fear seemed ridiculous, especially when I compared my output to Mozart and Beethoven.

Still, I loved the creative process. When I sat down and focused my troubled, chaos-filled mind on drawing or playing the piano, the physical sensation that resulted was similar to flying. Something happened deep within me and it felt like I was floating inside my body. The pleasure of watching what my hand would create and then how my mind would gently guide it onward toward some idealized goal was absolute bliss. It was as though my hand were dancing, trying its best to please my eye.

Because my parents wouldn't allow me to sleep outside in our stable, I was a closet dweller for much of my childhood. Like our backyard and the tack room, closets were my safe haven. One afternoon I happened to notice how large the closet of the bedroom I shared with Elaine looked. Not long afterward, I began begging my mother to let me relocate there and the next thing I knew she'd driven to Montgomery Ward and purchased a cot and a foam rubber mattress. I quickly shoved all my belongings inside, piled them sloppily into a corner, and shut the heavy wooden French doors. A single bare bulb dangling from the ceiling lit the place.

I remember feeling like Cinderella back then. Not so much because I thought my prince would someday appear; it was more because I considered my sisters evil. But they never bothered me in my closet. They left me alone in there to do the strange, misunderstood things only I had a knack for doing so well. My favorite pastime was rummaging through my toy box, looking for something to take apart, which was what I eventually did with all my toys. Everything I acquired, I dissected and never bothered to put back together again. Once, I found a box of straight pins and poked them through the eyes of my Barbie and Skipper dolls. When I emerged from my lair and showed them to one of the neighborhood kids, her mother grew angry with me, claiming I was a sadistic little girl.

"It's the only humane thing to do," I explained as she tried to shoo me out of her house. "Pupils are supposed to let the light in. But Barbie and Skipper didn't have pupils. Not real ones. They were only painted on."

I soon put those straight pins to good use. One morning, curled up on my cot, I began sticking myself with the pins and came to the conclusion that there was no sensation of pain between the first and second layer of skin. By the time Elaine pulled open the French doors, I'd stuck nearly all the pins in the box into the skin on my hands, arms, and legs.

My closet quickly became more than a place to sleep; it was my classroom. We had a swimming pool at our house and one time I pulled out the strainer and discovered dozens of lifeless beetles floating in the dirty water. I scooped them up, carried them back into my "bedroom," then managed to locate a piece of cardboard. Over the next half hour I painstakingly impaled each of the insects with pins and neatly arranged them on the cardboard, which I propped up against the wall. I thought it gave the place a certain museum feel.

"Come and look at my bug collection," I shouted while running around my neighborhood.

By the time we arrived back at my makeshift museum, something became horribly clear. The beetles had only temporarily drowned. Since I'd been out rounding up viewers, they'd come back to life and were now writhing grotesquely on the cardboard, helplessly attempting to escape. The neighborhood kids screamed and ran away.

Every lost soul has its Virgil, its guiding angel. I had Kerrie. She showed up one afternoon while I was sitting by myself in the spider-filled drainage pipe that ran underneath the highway in front of her newly built home.

When I first spotted her, she was marching toward my hiding place. Without a moment's hesitation, I started running in the opposite direction. From everything I knew about them at school, I didn't trust girls. In fact, I hated them.

"Hey," Kerrie shouted. "Come back here right now or I'm going to beat you up!"

I stopped dead in my tracks. She marched up to me and introduced herself. Even though she was a year older than me, we were soon inseparable at recess. Depending on who got out of class first, I'd either be waiting outside her classroom door or she'd be waiting outside mine. One of the things I liked about Kerrie was that she was tough as nails. She was the first person, besides my older siblings, who ever pummeled me in a fight. Her father trained her in the art of self-defense. She was the kind of girl who would sucker punch you for no reason. I'd never met anyone like her.

I was a strong child, familiar with using my fists at the drop of an insult or threat. This kept me quite busy and in fairly good fighting shape. But I relied more on my savage fury than tactics. Kerrie changed that. She taught me all about strategy. Rule number one: don't even think about attempting to fight her. Rule number two: when you punch, keep your thumb outside of your fist or you could end up breaking it.

Kerrie possessed the tight, efficient fighting style of a Golden Gloves boxer. When I threw a punch, I expended far too much energy and consumed entirely too much time with my sloppy swing. Her punches were swift and direct, with no wasted movement or energy. Yet there was also a softness to her. I always thought of Kerrie as a young lady tomboy. She had a sense of style and loved wearing hot pants or minidresses with bloomers underneath. She constantly berated me for not getting on my mother about the pathetic clothes she stuck me in. Strangely enough, my mother began listening to me when I told her I was sick of dressing like an inbred sharecropper. She started ordering me pleated skirts from the Sears, Roebuck catalog. One day, she even surprised me with a pair of fishnet stockings.

Besides changing the way I dressed, Kerrie also cured me of my propensity toward infantile play. One afternoon, she showed up at our house to find me crawling on the floor, sucking my thumb. Standing over me like a short-tempered drill sergeant, she shrieked, "Quit acting like a dork!" As harsh as her words were, nobody had ever cared enough about me to hit me with such a constructive scrap of criticism. She was absolutely right. I was acting like a pathetic dork. And when she shouted that at me, I felt like someone was holding a mirror in front of me, allowing me to see myself for the first time. That was the day I stood up and never again crawled around on the floor like a baby.

I began spending as much time as I could at Kerrie's genteel and well-mannered house. Everyone seemed to follow a set of clear-cut rules. I loved that. Her mother would quietly show me how to sit at a table and eat in a civilized fashion, instead of like a wild animal. She'd gently touch my dirt-smeared arm whenever I made some infraction. I soon learned to watch her closely and I began to imitate her slow, deliberate, polite movements at the table. For me, meals had always been a time where I'd cram as much food into my mouth as possible. I never dared utter a word. Because I was normally the butt of everyone's jokes, the moment I'd satisfy my hunger, I'd literally flee outside or disappear into my closet. That never happened at Kerrie's kitchen table. We'd actually sit around discussing the environment, politics, or art.

When Kerrie first punched her way into my life, I'd actually become a pretty good student. My downward spiral hadn't yet occurred. In fifth grade I scored so high on the battery of standardized tests we had to take that school officials made me retake it. They couldn't understand how someone my age could be reading and performing mathematical calculations at a high school level. I couldn't explain it either, especially my peculiar aptitude for math. My uncanny ability to always be able to choose the correct answer from the ones provided seemed so natural, almost like breathing. When they made me retake the test, they asked me to show how I had arrived at my answer on the math portion, a task that made everything much more difficult. Because when it came to solving mathematical problems, the answers literally just came to me. All I needed to do was supply my brain with the necessary raw material and it did the rest. I still scored in the top 2 percent.

By seventh grade, however, everything changed. At the time, I couldn't put my finger on why, but it scared me. My life as a wanderer began at that point. I floated from moment to moment, blown by the whim of whatever was going on inside my brain. I'd gone from being the smartest girl in my class to a hopeless drifter. Now I've come to understand that the reason for this shift was because the one safe, predictable part of my life had been turned upside down. All at once, I'd left the comforting cocoon of elementary school, where the classes were small and I often remained with the same teacher for the entire day, and entered the chaos of junior high. Trying to find my way from one class to the next, amidst all the noise and kids, was far too much for my delicate system.

Almost overnight I noticed that I just could no longer hold numbers in my head. In between the time I began inputting the information into my brain, then attempted to work out the problem on paper, the numbers would float away and evaporate. After awhile, I convinced myself that I was becoming mentally retarded and fell into a dark depression. I missed the safety of having a single teacher who taught me all my subjects, often someone who took me under her wing and served as a mentor. Sometimes it almost felt like I was floating away, drifting into space, and there was nothing I could do to root myself back into the ground. Clearly, my Asperger's was beginning to blossom inside me in a way that not even I could ignore.

Before long, Kerrie became my only friend, a fact she used to wield over me like a razor-sharp machete. She ordered me to do things and I was powerless to tell her no. Her favorite pastime was to have me follow her to her boyfriend's house, then instruct me to watch their make-out sessions. The two of them would smoke Mexican pot as I sat there on the floor, watching them kiss and fondle each other. It bored me senseless, but I felt like I had no choice in the matter, like I somehow had become trapped inside a web so vast and desolate that I'd never be able to muster up the strength necessary to escape. I was doomed. I could feel it deep in my gut.

Whenever the urge would hit her, Kerrie would hurl insults at me and I'd just sit there and take it. "I'm much prettier than you are," she'd scream while her boyfriend sucked a hickey into her neck. "Everyone says that." A moment later she'd whisper: "You know, my legs are much more beautiful than yours." I'd just nod passively. After years of feeling nothing but loneliness, I told myself that her verbal abuse was a small price to pay for the luxury of having someone pay attention to me.

By the beginning of ninth grade, I began to suspect that my brain had melted. All day long, I'd sit at my desk staring at my teachers, unable to understand what they were saying. They'd open their mouths, but the only thing to come out were incomprehensible strings of sound. I became hopelessly lost. The only class I bothered to attend was music. After all, I played the piccolo in the school band, the string bass in orchestra, and sang alto in chorus. The rest of the time, I'd wander off to a shady, secluded part of the school grounds and sit in the grass with the other kids cutting class. We'd play guitar and sing hippie songs. Sometimes we'd wander out into the desert and smoke pot or eat LSD and I'd stare up into the sky and wonder how long it would be before I lost it for good.

I didn't have to wait long to find out. The night I finally crossed over the line happened just after my parents had departed for a trip to India. In their place, they left an old family friend named Lester in charge of the kids. Lester was something of a country bumpkin who seemed to be the godfather to everyone in the family but me. Kerrie and I were sitting around at her house in ankle-length, psychedelic, green-and-purple paisley granny dresses when it dawned on me that it was time for me to return home. Lester would probably be worried.

"It's getting late," I announced.

"I'll walk you home," she replied.

The two of us made it as far as the mailbox in front of her house on Catalina Highway when Kerrie suddenly felt an idea overpower her.

"Here comes a car," she said. "Let's stick out our thumbs and see if they pick us up."

They did. A few minutes later we were five miles down the road at a tourist trap known as Trail Dust Town. We both knew someone who worked at the local ice cream shop there, so we dropped by and bummed a few free scoops, then walked back out to the strip of asphalt—still hot from being baked all day by the sun—that stretched out across the desert, back to our homes.

"Hey," Kerrie roared, "let's go to a bar."

It seemed like an awful idea, but I really wasn't looking forward to returning home. So we pointed our thumbs into the darkness. A single short ride later, we ended up at a sleazy bar and danced to the rock 'n' roll rumbling out of the scratchy jukebox. After a few hours, we hooked up with two bikers I vaguely recalled meeting several months before through my sister Barbara. They both had motorcycle chains wrapped around their hands, which I thought looked cute. They drove us back to their dirty apartment, filled us full of Gallo wine, then attempted to have sex with us. When they realized how drunk we were, they let us pass out on their couch. Kerrie vomited.

Things went downhill from there. The next morning, one of

our scraggly hosts suggested we embark on a road trip to Berkeley, a mythic place that every wannabe hippie and burnout in my
high school had been whispering about for the past year. So off we
roared across the Arizona desert. The first night of our odyssey, I
lost my virginity to a biker with a black patch over his eye, near a
rest stop in Oakland. He was a draft dodger trying to make his way
up to Canada. The night was foggy and we were crammed inside a
sleeping bag, lying in the dirt beneath a grove of eucalyptus trees.
I closed my eyes and sucked the moist, sweet air into my lungs. It
was unlike anything I'd ever experienced in dry, hot Arizona. I lay
there on my back with my one-eyed lover on top of me, staring up
at the outlines of the tree branches against the night sky. The pain
was exquisite, pure ecstasy. Somewhere in the back of my head, I
wondered if I was going to get pregnant. I was fourteen years old.

The next morning, I met back up with Kerrie at the rest stop.
"Well?" she asked, wanting to hear the sordid details of my de-
flowering. I just shrugged. I'd already put the whole episode
behind me.

"I've got an idea," I whispered. "We're in Oakland. Let's go see
the Black Panthers."

Kerrie smiled. We climbed back into the car. Its driver happened to be the same guy with the motorcycle chain wrapped
around his hand we'd met days before at that bar back in Arizona. I'd been fascinated with the Panthers ever since I'd smoked
opium and made out with a black boy from a rival high school a
few months before. Before I met him, I thought every kid had a
stable in their backyard. But after spending some time in the tiny
run-down apartment he shared with his mother and three sisters,
I began to understand how the rest of the world lived. Try as I
might, I just couldn't understand how people could hate an entire
race, especially when they had such nice, soft, kissable lips.

When we finally managed to locate the Black Panther headquarters in a tired-looking stretch of inner-city Oakland, they
didn't exactly look thrilled to see the three scraggly white kids

from Arizona standing in their front office. Four of the group's members stared at us, unsure of what they were looking at. They glanced at each other almost nervously. I held my fist in the air.

"Power to the Panthers!" I shouted. "Fight the Man."

Nobody smiled. Finally one of the men asked, "What are you doing here?"

"We drove here from Arizona," I replied. "We've heard all about you, so we wanted to meet you and see what you were all about."

"You did?" he replied coolly. "Now ain't that special?"

For what seemed like the next few minutes, nobody said a word. We all just stared at each other in silence. Finally, one of the Panthers announced, "Okay, you saw what we were all about. Now you best be moving on."

Afterward, when we got back in the car, I said, "I guess they don't get a lot of white people at Panther headquarters."

Kerrie shook her head angrily. "What a bunch of assholes," she mumbled before flying into a jealous rage over my confession that I'd actually had a black lover months before.

Our next stop was Berkeley, where my older sister Elaine was living in a '58 GMC panel truck, covered with her Day-Glo paintings of Charlie Brown smoking joints. She'd disappeared to Berkeley a few months before to riot, carouse, and try to make it as a psychedelic artist. The minute we arrived, I fell in love with the place—it was like a living, breathing organism filled with an army of misfits and castoffs just like me. All my life, I'd seen myself as an outsider, like everyone was watching and judging me, and no matter what I did I could never fit in. I could only pretend I did. But in those dirty streets of Berkeley, I felt like I belonged, like I no longer had to fake it. The sensation was intoxicating—even without all the drugs. I never wanted to leave. I wanted to rip my clothes off, throw back my head, and shriek with giddy ecstasy.

Within hours of arriving, Kerrie fell under the spell of a street hustler and moved in with him. Meanwhile, I was running around barefoot, smoking opium and marijuana, panhandling for food, making love with strangers, and sleeping on an old mattress in a basement with a bunch of runaways. I spent days sitting in front of a hippie poster shop hoping to run into Elaine. I figured that since she was an artist, she probably had some artwork hanging inside. A week later, we bumped into each other. She looked less than thrilled to see me, especially when she learned about my exploits over the past ten days. She immediately telephoned my mother, who was in Japan at the time. Two days later, she appeared in Berkeley with Kerrie's father and the four of us returned to Tucson.

"You know Lester had a heart attack," my mother explained coolly during the long, nearly silent flight home. "He's been worried sick about you. You're going to call him when we get home and apologize."

"Apologize? . . . For what?" I asked.

"For causing his heart attack, that's what," she snapped.

I felt terrible thinking that I'd caused Lester pain. And for a few fleeting moments, I wondered why it never dawned on me that he might be worried. Was I really that dense? But more than anything else, I was consumed by sadness. The dirty streets of Berkeley marked the first place I'd ever felt truly alive and accepted. Chaos becomes me, I thought, convinced I'd die if I didn't return.

CHAPTER FOUR

From somewhere on the other side of my bedroom door, I heard him approaching. I was sitting on my bed, this month's *Playboy* centerfold spread out below me. The sound my father's shoes made on the hallway floor resembled thunder. The brunt of the storm, I knew from similar experiences, would soon follow. Within seconds he would fling the door open and stomp inside. I didn't want to think about what would happen next. Too much left to do. I attempted to focus on the task at hand, but realized my concentration was slipping.

"Jerry!" my father shouted. "What in God's name are you doing in there?" Years would pass before I finally knew the answer to that question, before I ever understood anything about how to deal with a woman other than gawk at her nude body in a girlie magazine. Mary taught me that. She helped me to finally understand one of the most important lessons a man can ever learn—that a woman is much, much more than the sum of her parts. And that the first step toward treating a woman—or anyone, for that matter—with respect comes only when you learn how to treat yourself with respect. Mary taught me that lesson without ever saying a word.

But on that evening when my father roared that question at me, it took me a few moments before I understood that he actually wanted an answer. For as long as I could remember, rhetorical questions had always confused me. Why ask something if you already know the answer? I fumbled to conceal my activity, but I knew it was pointless. Heartbeats later, the door exploded open and my father was suddenly standing in my bedroom. His teeth were clenched, his lips taut. He glared at me. I dared myself to glance into his eyes, but I could do it for only a few moments. Then I turned away. What I glimpsed there confused me—a strange combination of anger, frustration, and sadness.

"Why do you want to do this?" he demanded. "Do you want to knock someone up? Is that what you want to do?"

I didn't know what to say, so I sat there mute, staring halfheartedly at the nude woman on my bed, feeling ashamed. I wanted to tell him how much it hurt when everyone teased me in the shower or in the men's room at the speedway, teased me about my anatomy. Over the past year, I'd convinced myself that there was something biologically wrong with me, some sort of physical glitch that was going to doom my chances of ever being with a woman. I wanted to tell him that my sessions with *Playboy* were my way of proving to myself that nothing was wrong with me, that everything was working just fine. But I didn't dare tell him any of that because it would only make him angrier. He clenched his right fist, then relaxed it. I knew what came next. He charged at me, cocked back his right arm, and slapped me in the face. Not hard, but hard enough.

"This isn't a good thing to be doing, Jerry!" he shouted. "I never want you to do this again."

He slammed the door behind him with such force that the whole house shook. I sat there, slumped over, not bothering to look up, just wanting to cry. So much for playing with my erector set. I folded up the centerfold, closed the magazine, then shoved it under my mattress, promising myself I would never do this again. But I knew I would probably be right back at it tomorrow night after dinner.

Masturbation was all I had and now I felt guilty about it. My friends had girlfriends. They could walk up to a girl they thought was cute and talk to her about anything that came to mind. But not me. I was so painfully shy and awkward around the opposite sex that my classmates went out of their way to tell me not to attend their parties. "No-Newport parties," I'd begun calling them. I made the other kids nervous, the way I lurked around by the punch bowl, desperately attempting to strike up a conversation with anyone who strayed into my vicinity.

I had crushes on a few girls in my class, but they never amounted to anything. They always chose the other guy. I never even mustered the courage to let a single one of them in on what was going on inside my heart. My need to acquire a girlfriend reminded me of the time when I was six and I ran all over our neighborhood trying to catch a butterfly. The funny part was, I didn't know what to do with it when I finally cupped one within my hands. To make matters worse, my middle brother, Jim, had been going on dates since he was in seventh grade. When I won the county math contest, I cooked up this fantasy about taking my trophy and giving it to Judy, on whom I had my first real crush. Her response? She tossed it out the window and told me that what she really wanted was a baseball trophy, like the one her boyfriend, Don, won every year as one of the school's top pitchers.

When it came to navigating social situations, everything felt shrouded in an impenetrable mist. I felt so disoriented, so confused about where to take my next step that all I could do was stumble pathetically. I needed some sort of compass, some kind of a guide. I kept asking myself, How does everyone else know what to do? Did they read about it in a book somewhere? I needed someone to talk to, someone with answers or just a few helpful suggestions about how to proceed.

But it was so tough for me to give up control like that, to actually admit to someone that there were questions I didn't have all the answers to. It has taken me a lifetime to try to overcome that character trait, although I think I've finally convinced myself that there are plenty of things I don't know and I'm actually okay with it. It no longer sends me into a panic when it hits me that there are facts and equations floating around out there in the universe that I haven't mastered. But back then in school I was the one with all the answers. Not that I was really fooling anyone, though. And God knows my parents didn't even want to think about what I was going through. As far they were concerned, whatever I was doing up in my room after dinner was perverted, wrong, and would only lead to one thing—my turning into a sex maniac, knocking up some girl, then having a shotgun wedding. But I didn't care. Masturbation had become my only release. The imagined relationships I had with the women in the pages of *Playboy* for a brief instant almost seemed real. The fog I'd been wandering through would suddenly lift, and I'd find someone out there who could look into my confused heart and understand everything going on inside of me. She accepted me better than I accepted myself.

While I pretended to be having sex with the glossy Playmate, what I truly yearned to be doing was talking to her. I wanted someone I could open up my heart to, someone who would listen to all things going on inside me and not judge me for it. Which wasn't to say that I couldn't converse with members of the opposite sex. In fact, when I was serving as the manager for the Islip High School basketball team I had gabfests with some of the school's most beautiful, popular young women. Yet, for all the words we exchanged with one another, the only thing we spoke about was idle gossip. The most beautiful of the bunch was Marianne, a sweet-natured junior who had caught the eye of nearly every member of the junior varsity and varsity teams. During away games I'd often sit on the bus next to Marianne and a gaggle of other cheerleaders, and we'd talk about who was going to end up together at that night's after-party. They were some of the most popular girls in the school, all of whom dwelled in a completely separate social dimension from me, located so many light-years beyond my world that I didn't even bother fantasizing about them. But the more I got to know them, the more I sat on that bus listening to their fears and fantasies, the more I understood why I never got tongue-tied around them.

They were freaks, just like me. Only their freakishness was due to their exquisite physical perfection, their long, slender legs, their well-organized faces with noses that turned up just so and their perfectly shaped eyes. I was simply a freak because I was a math geek, a human computer with the unnerving habit of picking his nose at the most inappropriate moment, then popping the gooey morsel into his mouth, chewing it up, and swallowing it. Yet, in our own ways, we both felt like museum specimens, caged oddities. The kids at school gawked at them for all the right reasons. They stared at me for all the wrong reasons. Either way, it was still draining to know that the moment you walked onto the school grounds, you were there for everyone else's entertainment. Sitting with Marianne and her friends, I felt a sense of acceptance that I never experienced with the general population of our school.

And acceptance was something I craved. More than anything else, I yearned to be one of the guys. I would have gladly traded my gift with numbers for the ability to walk, converse, and think like everyone else, for the priceless ability to make small talk. So far, the only thing my uncanny propensity toward number crunching had earned me was a handful of trophies and medals from various math contests organized by a local actuary society and a spot on the school's math team. Even there, I spent most of my time on the bench because the teacher who served as the coach only wanted to use her senior number whizzes, despite the fact I could leave them in the dust when it came to crunching math problems. It never dawned on me that our coach was just trying to help her seniors polish their skills so they could perform better on the SATs and get into college.

I was fifteen years old when it finally dawned on me that I was looking for acceptance in all the wrong places. My parents had left me alone for the night while they went to see a movie. I invited a bunch of my would-be buddies over to hang out at my house. Most of these guys had girlfriends who were away at the same slumber party; I figured they probably had nothing better to do. Within minutes of arriving, they fanned out through our house, executing a well-planned campaign of mayhem. They dumped my dad's shoes into my aquarium and set all the alarm clocks to go off for 3:00 a.m. One guy even emptied his bowels in the top drawer of my mother's dresser. When they discovered my brother's archery set in the garage, they soaked the arrows in gasoline, lit them, then shot them high into the black night sky. Before long, they fled into the night laughing, heading off to embark on a panty raid. I walked into our ransacked kitchen. My father had left a sign on the refrigerator: Help yourself to the food, but leave the cherry pie alone. On a nearby table sat the empty pie tin, its contents devoured several minutes before.

Sitting down beside the red-smeared metallic carcass, my mind was whirring. Why are you so desperate to hang out with these guys? Why is it so important for you to be with the in-crowd? Is it really worth all this abuse? I went to work cleaning up, then stumbled off to bed.

Not long after that I made a conscious decision to stop chasing a bunch of guys who never really liked me, but only tolerated me. And I found some real friends, late-bloomers like me, a smattering of socially inept geeks I knew from the math club, the school band, and Boy Scouts. We'd drive around the streets of Islip, throwing eggs, tipping trash cans, cruising the bowling alley and the local McDonald's parking lot, looking for any opportunity to create havoc. We also loved terrorizing our more popular classmates, the jocks and cool kids who actually had dates. Whenever we'd spot a car parked in some secluded locale, we'd kill our lights and quietly coast up behind the two lovebirds. It was never anything personal. In fact, we actually liked most of the people we were hazing. Nevertheless, tormenting them just felt like the right thing to do. We were both fulfilling our natural roles—they got to make out with one another and we got to harass them. Besides, the looks on their faces when we'd hit our headlights, lay on the horn, and began heaving eggs were worth all the harassment we'd receive the following Monday at school. And by the end of the week, all was usually forgiven.

Despite giving up on associating with the popular set, my best and longest-running friendship at school was with Johnny Aichroth, a gifted athlete, an excellent musician, a brilliant student, and an all-around good guy. Not long after the Friday night assault on our house, Johnny collapsed at wrestling practice. For the next few months he was shuttled from one hospital to another. Because he was such a well-liked kid, everyone would visit him, which drove the nurses crazy. They'd always shoo us out of his room until we figured out that we should pretend to be visiting other patients. In order to keep me from tipping off the nurses because I couldn't act or lie if my life depended on it, I always got to sit next to Johnny's bed. He looked gaunt and pale. The doctors were stumped.

"When you get out of here, I'll take you water skiing whenever you want next summer," I stammered. Johnny seemed to be slipping away before my eyes and nobody could do a thing about it.

"Sure, Jerry," he smiled, looking so undignified in the pathetic white smock they made him wear. "Jerry, you take care of yourself . . . okay?"

When Johnny died on Valentine's Day, 1964 (which happened to fall on a Friday), word moved through the town like a gust of bad wind, blowing from one end to the other. That morning, my father stopped me in the hallway and he didn't have to say a single word. His tears said everything I needed to know. I wandered into civics class, feeling numb, and whispered the news to Ted Herrmann, sitting behind me. Within minutes, Mr. Handler stopped his lecture to ask his sobbing class what had happened. That night, the high school basketball team dedicated the game to Johnny and won a major upset over a rival who had always decimated us. Graduates who had known Johnny journeyed back from college just to attend his funeral.

I felt the loss enormously. But I couldn't quite figure out what to do with all that alien emotion simmering inside me. Within the space of a calendar year, I had lost the three Johns in my life— Johnny; President John F. Kennedy, gunned down in Dallas the previous November; and my brother, John, who hadn't died, but had just grown up, graduated from college, and moved out of the house. Johnny's death bewildered me. When President Kennedy died, I sat through the memorial service at our church and cried my eyes out. But when one of my best friends died, I couldn't shed a tear.

At his burial, I stood in the background, far from all the other mourners, curiously watching how the sadness affected everyone, not sure what to make of any of it because I simply could not process the information. Yet at the same time I realized it should be affecting me, and that troubled me in a way I couldn't name. The kids from school encircled Johnny's grave, crying, holding hands, leaning on one another's shoulders. But I refused to allow myself to share my sadness with anyone. It seemed like the ultimate act of rebellion. As Johnny's best friend I was expected to display my grief to the community. But since I'd never felt like I was part of the community, I convinced myself that I wasn't going to let myself be recruited into their grief ritual. As if I actually had any say in the matter. And as they lowered Johnny's body into the cold dirt, I'd never felt quite so separate from the people around me, so sealed off, as though I'd been encircled by an impenetrable wall of concrete. I understood that the hurt that now consumed me was similar to everyone else's. The only difference was that I was alone with my sorrow. I could feel it rumbling around inside me. But it wouldn't come out. I had it all to myself.

By the time my senior year rolled around, I'd pretty much checked out from school. The summer before, I'd attended a seven-week camp that merged science and technology with the humanities at the Clarkson Institute, located three hundred glorious miles north of Islip. It was my father's idea. Years before, he'd become haunted by the story of a young mathematics savant who ended up graduating from Harvard while still in his teens. A hopeless social outcast without a single friend, he was consumed by subways and the knowledge that it was possible to ride the entire New York City subway system on a single token. He was in his early twenties when some strangers discovered him just minutes from death in a subway car. His last words were: "Goddamn my father!" Ever since the day he first heard that story, my father desperately did not want that to be my fate.

"Just being smart in math isn't enough," he'd always tell me. "You have to know how to communicate. You have to know how to write."

Those seven weeks away from home made me so bullish on what lay ahead for me in college that I didn't want to return to high school. It marked the first time I'd ever met so many kids who were academically superior to me. It was intoxicating. Several of them went on to become Rhodes scholars and National Merit scholars. Instead of sitting in class, waiting for the other kids to try to catch up with me, I was on my toes, my brain was on fire. Instead of extinguishing the blaze, the other kids poured on the gasoline and kept tossing lit matches.

Returning to Islip High School was almost more than I could bear. I counted the days until graduation. The only good thing to happen during my senior year was that I finally mustered up enough nerve to ask a girl out on a date. But instead of becoming a happy turning point in my life, the event was merely another sad example of my making a bad choice. Gloria was a freshman with a cute face, a quick wit, an ample chest, and the kind of reputation that I'd spent years fantasizing about. I took her to a lawn party. On the way there, we drank a few of the beers I'd convinced someone to buy for me. Upon arriving, I wandered off to use the bathroom and when I returned I found a group of guys had lined up in front of Gloria. They were waiting their turn to make out with her. I couldn't believe it. I stood there watching the strange scene as one person after another awkwardly kissed and groped her. After a few minutes, I decided to take my place in line to see if I could get in on the action. After all, she'd come to the party with me.

On our next date, Gloria disappeared shortly after we arrived at the party. I finally located her in the bushes with a guy from the basketball team. At least it wasn't a group effort this time, I told myself. Later that night, she and her new beau asked me to drive them home. They sat in the backseat while I navigated the streets of Islip. I was crying, but I don't think either one of them noticed. College couldn't come soon enough.

In addition to a handful of state schools, I applied to Harvard and Princeton. My father told me he'd buy me any car I wanted if I could actually get in, but it eventually became apparent that I wasn't going to be Ivy League material. It took only one alumni interview before I was sized up as someone who might actually be smart but definitely didn't have the social skills required to carry the crimson or orange banner.

I think my father and I were both relieved. He definitely couldn't afford the car. And I couldn't bear the thought of cruising up to Harvard in my new Corvette, then opening the door and stepping out wearing my pathetic Sears, Roebuck wardrobe. The day I got my acceptance letter from the University of Michigan, I'd already made up my mind to attend school there. I'd been intrigued by the place ever since I was in grade school, when my mother bought me a twelve-volume set of math books. Two of the texts, which dealt with topics like geometric inequalities and visual mathematics, were written by University of Michigan professors. I had imagined taking classes from them and quickly convinced myself that the university had the kind of math program that would be perfect for me. But its biggest appeal was the number of miles that Ann Arbor, Michigan, was located from Islip—seven hundred. The distance not only seemed just large enough to prevent my parents from visiting every weekend, but it also would keep any of my classmates from applying there. That was important to me. Because more than anything else, I yearned to go somewhere and start afresh. I told myself that would be the only way I'd ever be able to find *new* friends, *real* friends. And I dreamed about the day I'd return home to Islip with my new girlfriend clutching my arm and make everyone in town feel awful for not treating me better.

After what seemed like a lifetime, my graduation finally came. Since I had the second-highest GPA in my class, I was granted the honor of delivering the salutatorian address, during which I railed and ranted against the evils of nepotism and our culture's sheep-like tendency to follow hairstyle and clothing trends. Instead of my normal monotone, my voice felt animated, electric, packed with inflection. Unfortunately, my impassioned rant didn't go over exactly as planned. The audience, which had packed into our sweltering high school gymnasium, just watched me nervously. When it was over, no one applauded. Not that I gave a rat's ass. I was so over high school, Islip, and living at home that the only thing I wanted was to be gone.

"Helluva speech, Newport," my pal Steve told me afterward. "Never knew you were so angry at the world."

"Yeah, it sorta came out that way, didn't it?" I mumbled.

"Forget about it," he insisted. "Come on, let's go get some beers before the senior dance."

"I'm not going," I announced.

"What?" he stammered. "Everyone's going."

I didn't even bother replying. I just walked out into the humid summer night and headed home. All I wanted to do was lock my bedroom door, flop down on my bed, and zone out in the comforting cathode glow of my TV. Maybe, if I was lucky, I'd be able to catch a rerun of my favorite show, *The Untouchables*. The irony of it all went right over my head.

SOMEWHERE BETWEEN MINGUS AND RANGER, TEXAS
MARCH 1970

Sitting in the backseat of the rental car, I watched as the rickety wooden fence posts flickered and flashed past my window like rows of nicotine-stained teeth. My parents didn't utter a word, only bothering to crack open their lips when they needed to breathe through their mouths. So we rolled across the scraggly, hilly countryside of west Texas like three mutes, speeding toward my new home at the Children of God compound located in a muddy ghost town. All roads led to there. After returning from my odyssey in Berkeley with Kerrie, I'd been sent to live with my sister Carolyn and her husband, Keith, in Tucson. I just ended up taking more blotter acid, smoking more pot, and having lots of sex.

Jerry did his share of drugs in the sixties, but they didn't mess with his head quite the way they did with mine. He's more stable in that way. His mind tends to be much better anchored in that firmament that roots us to the here and now. I've always admired that about Jerry, always wished he could teach me that wonderful skill of remaining in the present. It certainly would have come in handy in my life. I suppose, however, that's not a skill you can teach someone, no matter how much you love and care for them.

But enough with all the reveries. On that humid morning, I was a few days away from my fifteenth birthday and an outcast.

Marjorie and Dr. Meinel were finally getting rid of me. I wondered how I felt. It certainly seemed like I should be experiencing some sort of emotion right about now. I told myself I should be relieved that I wasn't being shipped off to a mental institution like the one I'd heard rumors my parents were considering. But I certainly didn't feel relieved. I felt ... *nothing*. Whenever I reminded myself about what was happening, it seemed like a strange dream taking place inside someone else's head. Were the LSD trips catching up with me? Something had gone a bit wrong within my brain. Had my hallucinatory excursions to the other side of the universe fried my neural circuitry, leaving me unable to accurately perceive moving objects? Everything appeared strobelike and animated, confusingly surreal. Even worse, thoughts and emotions came to me in disjointed bursts. I'd become a walking zombie.

"There it is, Aden," I heard my mother say, pointing to a ramshackle clump of buildings on the horizon. "Up there ... look."

Moments later we pulled off the highway, into the decrepit remains of what once was a booming oil town that now resembled a bombed-out concentration camp. The ground had been sucked dry of oil. All that remained was mud. I started laughing. *This* was just too much. A man with a walkie-talkie and a ridiculous smile slogged his way through the earthy brown morass to our car. My mother curtly told him who we were. He nodded, whispered a few words into his walkie-talkie, then motioned for us to get out of the car. He introduced himself to us by his "Biblical" name—David Zebulon. The Children of God, he informed us, had been awaiting our arrival. For the next forty-five minutes he led us through the rich brown muddy clay, from one run-down building to the next.

"This is where you'll live," David Zebulon said, pointing inside a tiny building made from rough-hewn stones precariously stuck together by concrete. A single, endless row of bunk beds stretched across the room.

My sister Barbara, now known as Naomi, was working in the

nursery. She greeted us with the same blissed-out smile as our guide, who was whispering our every single movement into his walkie-talkie. My parents gave the place a quick once-over, although the tight-lipped, annoyed expressions on their faces convinced me that they wished they hadn't. All they wanted to be was gone from there, and I didn't really blame them.

When they finally climbed back into their rental car, I stood there watching them. Just before roaring off down the highway, my mother rolled down the window and leaned out. "Be good," was all she said. The next thing I knew, I turned around and began slogging my way through the mud, stumbling to the top of a hill above the compound. I sat down on the wet grass, wrapped my arms around my knees, and pulled my legs up tight against my chest. My parents were gone. They'd finally managed to rid themselves of me. I started to feel an emotion that resembled . . . *rejection* welling up inside my chest. But then a faint whisper inside my head reminded me that I was also rejecting them. That made me feel better.

Over the next few days, I began wondering why I'd ever decided to come. I'd known about the Children of God for several years, back when I sometimes played guitar with some members in a park near our house and they'd sing these hippie-style songs about Jesus. Barbara had decided to become a member, and by the time I began my long, downhill slide into drugged-out delinquency, she'd convinced the members to write me letters, telling me how much they loved me and wanted to help me. Whispers and rumors had begun circulating that my parents were considering sending me on an extended stay to a mental institution, something even they didn't want to do. When it finally became apparent that no boarding school wanted anything to do with a hard-luck case like me, I began to consider the group's offer seriously.

But the reality was different from what I remembered. The trippy, anything-goes hippie mentality had been replaced by one of extreme paranoia. Jesus still loved us, but the rest of the world obviously wanted to persecute us. I was told that to leave the compound property was the equivalent of committing suicide. The minute you set foot on the highway that stretched past our property, the gun-crazed rednecks who lived in the vicinity would blast you with shotguns. Before long, I grew deathly afraid of the outside world. Our leader was a charismatic, often moody man with an affinity for dark glasses, named David Berg. Somewhere along the way, he decided to call himself Moses, because he firmly believed he was leading the chosen few out of a corrupt, modern-day Egypt. He loved filling us full of stories—the Antichrist was lurking in our midst. The world would soon end. Dark forces would soon take over. Christians everywhere would be jailed and tortured. Unspeakable, horrific things lay in store for our tiny group of believers. Death was a certainty.

Most of my waking hours were spent praying, learning the Scripture from the books of Daniel and Revelation, and preparing for my martyrdom. Instead of finding acceptance, nearly everyone seemed either to hate me or, at best, be extremely annoyed by my presence. I tried to distance myself from their wrath, gathering up all their negativity, rolling it up into one giant black cloud, and moving it as far away from me as I could. No need to dwell on it. I was here for the long haul. After a month, my parents signed documents that granted the cult legal custody of me. At the time, my main duty involved rummaging through the crates of rotten vegetables that other members had pulled from Dumpsters in surrounding towns. Trying to find something edible in the slimy, gelatinous ooze was nauseating work. What once had been spinach, tomatoes, lettuce, and cabbage had been reduced to a foul-smelling liquid. I spent hours digging maggots out of potatoes and cutting out the rancid, rotten spots as though they were tumors. We'd stir our slop into the bubbling vats of chicken feed that had been purchased in fifty-pound sacks from a nearby animal feed store. It was our typical breakfast.

"This is . . . so gross," the other girls would whisper, clearly sickened by the sight of decomposing vegetables. Their prudish reaction always gave me a perverse chuckle.

"You ever killed a rattlesnake and eaten it?" I'd ask. "This isn't so bad. . . . You can actually eat the slime and not get sick, unless it's full of bacteria."

One morning, just as I was about to wade into a particularly foul-smelling box filled with some shapes that vaguely resembled cauliflower, I was informed that our leader had just been given a message from God that I needed to be married off to another Children of God member, whose *nom de cult* was Asaph of Abdullam. He always referred to himself as "Ace of All Trades." He was nineteen. I was sixteen. I'd only met him once before, while seated across from him at a meal, and the disgusted look on his face made it quite clear that he couldn't stand me. He couldn't understand why God would want to punish him by making him marry me.

"What did I do to deserve you?" he'd moan. "What did I do?"

But since he considered himself a lifer in the cult, he dutifully obeyed his order. I loved his thick eyebrows and his high cheekbones. Shortly after our marriage, he became the cult's official photographer, partly to get away from me. He always refused to take my picture, claiming my image was too ugly to capture on film. When we had sex, I wanted to cry. That was when it hurt the most to be with someone who hated me. But I knew that to refuse Asaph was to betray God and our leaders.

By the time I felt his child growing inside my belly, it had become apparent that America was on the brink of annihilation. The Antichrist was preparing to strike. So, the Children of God packed up and moved their operations to a shabby warehouse in Bromley, a suburb of London.

After insulting the daughter of the cult leader who had recently crowned herself the Queen of the Kingdom of God at a lavish coronation (she apparently didn't like being corrected on a bit of Old Testament trivia), I'd become something of a pariah in our commune. Everyone left me alone, which was heaven for me. I loved isolation and spent much of my time reading the Bible, trying to develop my spiritual powers. I still believed in God, but I had an unshakable hunch that He or She had nothing in common with the deity to whom my fellow cult members were praying. As far as theology was involved, I was simply going along for the ride—although I sometimes got caught up in the scenery rolling past the windows. During those days, I lived in a run-down house and tended to the commune's littlest members in the upstairs nursery. The only time I ventured outside the house was to proselytize to strangers, hawking Jesus to the unwashed masses. I was a rotten saleswoman for two reasons. I still struggled to communicate. I also was always too interested in what was going on inside the heads of my potential converts, which meant that I ended up letting them do most of the talking. My continual failure to bring any new members into the cult only added fuel to the rage directed against me.

It rained nearly every day. We didn't believe in doctors or modern medicine, so I suffered from a perpetual case of bronchitis and a constant earache. I was told that the pus dripping out of my ears was a visible reminder of my transgressions against God. I often sat in the nursery, staring through the rain-smeared window at the rooftops, enjoying the blurry, soft-focused visuals, frightened that I might be experiencing an acid flashback. I sang and played guitar for the infants and toddlers, trying to coax them into smiling or making their little eyes light up, trying to keep them from being as miserable as their parents were. Whenever I could, I'd attempt to communicate with the baby growing inside of me. I'd hum the song "You Gotta Be a Baby to Get into Heaven" and recite the story about the Pied Piper of Hamlin to whoever was living within my belly. Whether it was a boy or a girl didn't really concern me. I just knew that for the first time in my life, I was finally going to have someone in my life who loved and accepted me unconditionally—just as I was going to accept him or her unconditionally.

It was just around the time that I finally located a box of Q-Tips and secretly began using them to clean the infection out of my ears that we moved to our newest location—a winery in Basetto, Italy, just south of Florence. A Catholic duke had become one of our newest converts. The fact that he was Catholic—and remained so—could easily be overlooked because of his land holdings. I had just finished cooking breakfast for thirty of my "brothers and sisters" when my water broke. By then, Ace of All Trades had become infatuated with Barbara and somehow managed to convince the cult leaders to send him to France, where my sister was living with some other members. When our resident midwife, Keturah (named after Abraham's concubine) tried to check the state of my cervix with her fingers, she grew angry.

"God is not pleased with you," she hissed. "Your cervix ... it's located too high up for me to reach."

She begrudgingly telephoned a midwife who lived in a nearby village. She took one look at me writhing on top of my bed and announced in broken English that she could do nothing for me. I needed to be rushed to the local hospital.

"We don't do that," Keturah replied sternly. "We always have our births at home. We don't use hospitals."

The woman shooed Keturah away as if she were a pigeon. This made me smile. A few minutes later we were flying over the twisting roads of Poggibonsi in her tiny, battered Fiat. The hospital was run by nuns, who quickly pulled me from the car and wheeled me into the emergency room. Something about their eyes told me that I was in serious trouble. The pain was unlike anything I'd ever experienced. I slowed my breathing, pulling the stale antiseptic air of the hospital in through my nose, and recited a verse from the Book of Proverbs—"Great peace have they which love Thy law and nothing shall offend them." I wasn't afraid of death. It couldn't be any worse than life. If God wanted me to return home, I was ready to go.

A doctor gave me the once-over and ordered them to take

X-rays. The last thing I remember is hyperventilating wildly as Keturah argued with the doctor, insisting that X-rays weren't necessary. Deep down, I knew she didn't care one way or another if my baby lived or died. She'd let God make the call. "Let me take her back with me . . . back with me . . . back with me!" she screamed.

I woke up the next day in a room filled with women from the local village, lying in beds all around me. "Dolore . . . dolore . . . dolore," they moaned, asking for deliverance from their pain. I prayed that God would give them a hand. When they noticed my eyes were open, they smiled and shook their heads. No one could believe I was alive. My bronchitis had grown into full-blown pneumonia. Whenever I dared cough to clear my lungs, the enormous incision snaking up my belly erupted with spasms of pain. After a few minutes, a nurse arrived clutching my baby boy. He was the most beautiful thing I'd ever seen in my life. My heart felt on the verge of bursting. Within a split second, he became the only thing I cared about. My precious tiny gem. I laid him on my chest and watched his eyes flutter shut; then he drifted off to sleep with a microscopic smile on his face. I knew that he didn't care that everyone hated me, that everyone thought me a freak. Finally, I'd found someone who loved me as much as I loved him. I'd never felt anything like this before. It didn't even matter that the nurses refused to give me any painkillers or medicine. The emotion pouring out from my heart made my wounds and sickness dissolve.

Ace dropped by the hospital a few days later. He was clearly annoyed at having to leave France in order to come visit me. "God is punishing you," he said. "You know that, don't you? You're the first member to have a baby in a hospital. . . . You know how that makes me look?"

I nodded, truly feeling sorry for him. He never wanted to marry me, and now look at all the trouble I was causing him. I tried to cheer him up by getting him to hold his child. But he just looked at him as if he were an insect. "His name will be Stefano," he announced. It seemed like the perfect name. Not because I liked the sound of Stefano, which I actually hated, but because it reminded me of Stevie Weinstein, a childhood friend from Tucson who I used to love playing Bugs Bunny and Three Stooges with. From that day onward I called my baby Steve.

I remained in the hospital for nearly two weeks. Even though I never spoke a word to my roommates, it quickly became apparent to them that Steve had no clothes. Keturah had stolen them and refused to give them back. One day, an old woman showed up in my room with a bag full of beautiful hand-crocheted baby clothes, along with bottles of mineral water. Her gifts were the first kindness I'd experienced in years.

Not long after I returned from the hospital with Steve, Ace convinced the cult leaders to let him divorce me. My inability to bring new converts into the group proved I was a bad person. But for Ace, my greatest transgression was the C-section I'd had. My scar was a sign from God, a visible reminder of my unworthiness. Ace wanted to get as far away from me as he could. I eventually learned that I was being sent back to America. The rest of the group would soon be boarding a jet and flying to the North African nation of Libya. The country's leader, an army colonel named Mu'ammar Gadhafi, had fallen under the spell of our mercurial leader and invited him and his followers to live there. Despite the fact that America would soon be overtaken by the Antichrist, returning home seemed like a better option than moving to Libya. The afternoon Ace shoved my few belongings into a backpack and tossed it in the backseat of the group's battered black Fiat, I was ready. I wrapped Steve in a blanket, hopped inside the tiny car, and shut my eyes. Twenty minutes later, Ace pulled over to the side of the highway, leaned across me, pushed opened the car door, then tossed out my pack.

"Okay," he said. "This is a good place."

We were on the side of a highway, a few miles from the outskirts of Torino. "But I don't have any money, Ace—or diapers or food."

For the first time in his life, he actually smiled at me. This made his tiny mustache twitch. "Use your faith," he suggested. "Let it guide you. It's all you need."

Easy for him to say, I thought. He didn't have a nine-month-old child to care for. I climbed out of the car clutching Steve and gently kicked my backpack off the road, into the grass. Traffic whizzed by. Once again, I was cast out. Not even a cult of wackos wanted me. And once again, I felt a detached sense of acceptance. It was time to move on. After all, I desperately yearned to find God, but I sure as hell wasn't going to locate him by staying with a xenophobic, paranoid group like the Children of God. I bent down, picked up my pack, tossed it over my shoulder, and started walking up the highway, back toward America.

CHAPTER FIVE

ANN ARBOR, MICHIGAN
AUGUST 1966

The morning I staggered off the Greyhound onto the University of Michigan campus, a battalion of giant metal water sprinklers were beating out a rhythm that sounded wonderfully exotic. Nobody was up yet except for the gardeners. I'd ridden all through the night to get there, with my face pressed up against the window to look at the world blurring past. I've sometimes wondered if Mary ever got to take a bus ride like that, heading toward her future with a million butterflies flapping, trapped inside her stomach. I desperately want to believe she has. I want to know that in the midst of all her chaos, she's gotten to savor the same sweet moments of hope and promise that I have, like I tasted on that night ride. Because those are the things that stay with you in life, lighting the way when all you can see is darkness.

On that first morning at the University of Michigan, all I could see was wet grass as I tromped up toward a cluster of unfamiliar buildings that made me feel like I'd been transported to ancient Greece. Everywhere I looked, it seemed like massive white Greek columns were sprouting out of the ground. The air was already humid. I was sleepy, but my mind was churning away, trying to process the intoxicatingly alien world surrounding me.

From out of nowhere, I heard a tiny voice inside my head. Nobody knows you here. Nobody knows who you are. But by the time you leave, they will. Everybody around here will know Jerry Newport.

I kept walking, not quite sure where I was going. Not really caring. Everything here was fresh and new. I'd come for an education, but more than anything else I'd come to Ann Arbor with the idea of starting over, of re-creating myself. I wanted to bury the old Jerry Newport deep in the ground and forget about him. That was why I'd decided to go to college here. Every other school where I'd been accepted, somebody from my high school was attending. And they knew the Jerry I'd just killed and left behind— Jerry the freak . . . the social outcast . . . the guy who had all those problems with women . . . the walking, talking adding machine. I desperately wanted to avoid the scenario that had occasionally occurred in high school, the one where I'd meet some girl who knew nothing about my past, who seemed to be truly interested in me. That is until somebody I knew spotted the two of us talking and the next thing I knew he was telling her all about my strange numerical skills, trying to goad me into performing my tricks for her like some circus animal. That wouldn't happen here. Not if I could help it.

All I wanted to do now was blend in. I wanted finally to defeat that thing inside me that always made me so different, so out of sync with the world around me. My dad told me that one of the best ways to fit into the college scene was to join a frat. So when the fall rush parties kicked off, I attacked them with a fury, signing up for open houses at fifteen fraternities. My dad had been a Phi Delt, so they were on the top of my list. Unfortunately, I wasn't on the top of theirs. At their second rush party, one of the members put his arm around my shoulder and asked me to follow him.

"Hey, Jerry, come on upstairs for a moment," he said. I couldn't believe it. Were they really going ask me to join? From what I knew about the process, it definitely seemed a bit early in the game for that. But who knows? Maybe I'd made a good impression on them. A moment later, I was standing in one of the brothers' bedrooms. Four of the guys sat on a sofa before me, looking uncomfortable.

"Look, Jerry," one of them said. "It's ... it's not that anyone here doesn't like you."

"Yeah," another member piped up. "You seem like a great guy."

"It just seems like," the first one added, "maybe there might be another house where you could fit in better."

They smiled solemnly and almost in unison ran their hands over their prickly crew cuts. One of the guys went back to attempting to light his pipe. I was escorted downstairs and politely ejected into the night. Over the next few days, I learned that when it came to getting blackballed, the Phi Delts were actually a fairly humane bunch. At one frat house, I caught a brother inspecting the label on my overcoat, then frowning to another member when it became clear that my mother had purchased it at Sears, Roebuck. A few minutes later, I was shown the door.

But not all my rejections were due to the judgments of others. Often, I had no one to blame but myself. At one house, I was pulled aside after some of the members heard me going into graphic detail of the adventures I'd recently had with a freshman nursing student I'd met at their previous rush party. Deep down, I knew my bragging was inappropriate, but once I started recounting my conquest I just couldn't stop the words from tumbling out of my mouth. Two of the members just rolled their eyes when they heard my monologue. A few minutes later I was invited upstairs and told to take a seat.

"We know rush must be a new thing to you," I was told. "And we think you've got a future in the Greek system."

"Unfortunately, it's not with us," snapped his fellow henchman.

It didn't take long before I garnered a reputation, not unlike the one I'd earned in high school, for being socially clueless. Once classes started, I struck up the nerve to ask out a girl named Becky in my honors math class. She said yes. Not long afterward, I took her to a movie and, when the night was over, I received the customary thank-you peck on the cheek. In the weeks that followed, I repeatedly asked her out, but she always politely claimed to be busy. Before long, she stopped coming to our math class, yet I continued to telephone her, always asking for a date, always getting turned down. One afternoon, a guy I recognized as living on another floor of my dorm stopped by my room. His name was David.

"Hey, Jerry," he said, looking a bit uneasy. "We gotta talk."

"About what?" I asked.

"You ever wonder why Becky dropped out of your math class?" he queried.

"Not really," I replied.

"She's trying to avoid you," he said. "She's getting tired of you calling her, asking for dates." He tried looking me in the eye, but I avoided his gaze.

"What do you mean, she's trying to avoid me?" I stammered. "Why?"

"You know how many times you've called her, Jerry?" he asked. "Do you have any idea how many times?"

"A few, I guess," I said.

"Fourteen times," he replied. "In the past two months you've called her fourteen times."

I suddenly felt uneasy, wondering how I could be so dense, incredulous that I had such little insight into my own head and what made me tick. I was also angry at myself for being so clueless, for causing so much discomfort to someone as nice as Becky. She certainly didn't deserve to be treated like that.

"Don't make it fifteen, Jerry," he said. "Don't call Becky anymore, okay?"

He started walking out of the room, then turned to see me

standing there, not moving, staring a hole into the floor, mentally pummeling myself for treating her as though she were some particularly complicated calculus problem. The way I'd always looked at it, if I wanted something badly enough, all I needed to do was roll up my sleeves, focus my brain, and bust my ass; then I'd achieve my goal. Suddenly, it occurred to me that people weren't anything like calculus problems.

Why had it taken me so long to realize that?

"You know what my rule is, Jerry?" he asked.

"Huh, what?" I mumbled, trying to snap out of my introspective funk.

"My rule of dating," he said. "You know what it is? I call it my 'Law of Three Strikes.' If I get turned down for a date three times, I'm out. Time to move on."

I stood there, trying to swallow this simple pearl of wisdom. Why hadn't I thought of that before? Why hadn't anyone ever bothered to tell me that before? Besides the advice that Johnny's father gave me before his son died—about always wearing my rubbers before going wading—this was the best morsel of social etiquette I'd ever received.

"See ya 'round, Jerry," David said, disappearing down the hallway. I kinda wanted to hug him—that is, if I wasn't so allergic to hugs.

I eventually joined Delta Chi, a fraternity filled with the kind of guys who reminded me of my high school math team. I'd been holding out for an offer from a cooler house. But as the weeks passed and the rush parties continued, I kept thinking back to that night in high school when all those popular guys I desperately wanted to accept me trashed my parents' house. Even though it felt like it happened light-years ago, the taste that night left in my mouth was awful. Nearly everyone at the Delta Chi house was majoring in some sort of science-related field, which meant I could go

Greek and geek at the same time. I felt safe there amid the social ineptitude. Nevertheless, a true sense of intimacy existed in our house. Unlike other fraternities I'd come to know before getting blackballed, I felt my new brothers actually cared for one another.

By my sophomore year, our house—along with plenty of others on campuses around the nation—was in serious trouble. The antiestablishment movement sweeping the country made fraternities seem like an uncool waste of time. And in the fall of 1967, with no new pledges, our relatively tiny thirty-member house was on the verge of going under. That didn't sit well with me. If that happened, how on earth could I fulfill my master plan of re-creating myself? Suddenly, the survival of Delta Chi became crucial to my survival. I threw myself headfirst into the task, eventually running for frat president. People agreed to vote for me because I was so energetic in my quest to keep our house alive. But they also felt that I was desperate enough to kill myself if our house went under. They were probably right. I thought I'd cinched the position, until the day before the election, when one of my frat brothers stopped me in the back stairwell and confessed, "I don't really want to run for president. But something tells me that the only reason you want the post is because of your ego. That's not good for you or our house."

Steve was right, but my house voted for me anyway and I won by a handful of votes at the Monday night chapter meeting. I quickly found myself wishing that everyone had listened to my last-minute opponent. Before long, I was spending nearly every waking hour on a frenzied quest, trying to drum up new members for the house. I rarely studied anymore. My grades nose-dived. I succeeded in getting a handful of new pledges over the next two semesters, but I was an awful leader, completely unable to delegate authority. At our weekly meetings, I'd often get so flustered when my frat brothers would horse around, trying to disrupt things, that I'd fly into angry tantrums, pounding on the table, demanding they stop, screaming at the hecklers, attempting to restore order.

My fits were so hilariously funny—to everyone but me—that my frat brothers nicknamed me Rocky the Flying Squirrel in honor of the furry cartoon character popular on TV at the time.

One afternoon, in between classes, I walked over to the house for lunch. On my way to the kitchen, I passed a bunch of the guys sitting around in someone's bedroom, talking about me. They must have assumed I couldn't hear them, but I did. Instead of continuing on my way to lunch, I stood beside the door and listened.

"Good ol' Newport—our esteemed president," one of them said. "That guy is one big walking contradiction."

"He really thinks he's some sort of Don Juan," replied another voice.

"Hey, Newport can get a date with just about anyone," another voice added. "That guy has had more first dates than anyone on campus. Too bad they never lead anywhere."

"You don't suppose," queried yet another voice, "that ol' Newport is one of those idiot savants, do you?"

I'd heard enough. And what the hell was an idiot savant, anyway? I decided to skip lunch and make my way to the library, my favorite place for trying to score dates. After a few minutes of research, I located a back issue of *Look* magazine containing an article on savants and began thumbing through it madly. On page 116, I found it—a picture of some pathetic-looking guy in a straitjacket, snapped in a French mental institution. Sure enough, he could crunch numbers like a computer and perform tricks, like telling you on what day of the week someone was born after only learning someone's date of birth. My head started spinning. I told myself that there was more to me than just my uncanny knack for numbers. I shut the magazine, shoved it back on the shelf, and started walking the library aisles, trying to clear my head. The squeaking sound of my penny loafers echoed through the building, making a sound that resembled a yapping puppy. People looked up from their textbooks and smiled. Over the past few months, my habit of prowling the library in search of coeds while wearing those noisy loafers earned me the nickname Squeaky Shoes.

Something told me that my French counterpart would never be able to pull off such a feat. And that made me feel better. That made me feel like the two of us really had nothing in common except our ability to process numbers.

Whenever I spotted an attractive coed with her nose buried in a book, I employed an ingeniously simple technique that made use of my wonderfully superficial knowledge of just about any topic.

"Pardon me," I'd say. "I see you're reading a book on the French Revolution."

"It's for my history class," my target would explain.

"I've always been a big fan of Marie Antoinette," I'd reply. "You know I heard she didn't even speak French. She was Austrian."

"Really?" she'd ask.

"Yeah," I'd say. "Hey, maybe we could get a cup of coffee sometime. I'll give you the inside scoop on the French Revolution."

My strategy nearly always worked because my marks were so surprised that a guy might be interested in meeting them to discuss something intellectual, or at least that's what I always told myself. They almost always agreed to that cup of coffee. Of course, those first dates rarely led anywhere. Why on earth would they? I was still so insecure, so desperately unsure of what to do with a woman other than try to get her into bed, that every date began plotting her escape minutes after I picked her up.

"You better take me back to my dorm now," one woman politely told me after listening to me pontificate upon all my achievements and reasons why I was better than all the other guys on campus.

"Oh," I said, surprised, but perhaps not really, that she didn't want to listen to my vain monologue. "Okay ... sure."

We walked back to her dorm in silence. When she spotted the front door, she darted up ahead of me. But just before disappearing inside, she said something that nearly knocked me over. "You know, I could see where I might be able to like you," she told me. "But you've got a lot of growing up to do." She smiled at me, the kind of smile that felt so real and honest but at the same time made me feel like an idiot because, at that moment, I was anything but real and honest. Despite not wanting to endure another minute in my presence, she actually seemed to care about me. And those last few words she said to me hit me with the force of a baseball bat.

"And why don't you ever look anyone in the eye?" she asked.

I stood there, staring up at her on the top step of her dorm, unable to say a word. I wanted to run. For the first time all night, I'd been struck mute. I bit my lip to keep myself from crying. Up until that moment, I'd somehow convinced myself that no one noticed my inability to make eye contact because I'd become so skilled at covering it up. When speaking to someone, I either focused my gaze to the right of their face or squarely upon the center of their forehead. To dare look into their eyes, to even ponder it, was to risk overloading my brain with so much data that I'd end up forgetting my painstakingly rehearsed monologue. Other people's eyes were nothing but trouble. I didn't even try telling that to my well-intentioned date. I just shrugged and walked back to my frat house.

Women were the ultimate mystery to me. What made them so enigmatic was how they always managed to bring out my worst, most insecure behavior. Even when I managed to land a second date, I was often filled with so much self-doubt that my insecurity quickly cast a black shadow over the evening. For instance, if I arrived to pick up my date and she kept me waiting, I instantly assumed I'd been stood up. After five minutes, I'd be transformed into a nervous, disheveled, sweating wreck. And when she did show up, the woman would find me pacing back and forth, running my fingers through my hair, lost in a deep, dark funk.

The summer of 1968, I lost my virginity to a hooker in a tired old hotel in San Francisco while tripping on LSD. One Saturday night, not long after arriving back on campus, I had sex with a girl I'd met at a kegger. Afterward, I lay next to her and began pouring my heart out to her ... about another girl I'd actually gone on several dates with. I asked her for some advice about how to get this other girl to spend more time with me. It never dawned on me that I was acting like the ultimate insensitive rube. Not at first it didn't. That part of my brain didn't exist. One minute I was simply having awkward sex with a woman, the next my mind had drifted off to another woman. Instead of keeping those thoughts quiet and separate, like any normal person would have, I blurted out exactly what was going on inside my head.

Years later, I realized it was my Asperger's doing the talking—not me. But on that sad night, one hurtful word after another just kept tumbling out of my mouth. When it finally hit me that maybe I should shut up, it was too late. Like some runaway train, my words had built up too much momentum for me to put the brakes on. My date closed her eyes and made one of those I-wish-I-were-a-thousand-miles-away-from-here faces. She turned mute. After awhile I ran out of words and lay there beside her, feeling like an imbecile, staring out into my filthy, garbage-strewn room, wondering if she knew how lost I felt in the world.

"Take me home now," she demanded.

"Okay," I replied, hoping that maybe she'd kick me in the crotch, because I had a hunch I'd done something to deserve it. But all she did was get dressed and quietly walk out into the hallway and wait.

By the summer before my senior year, I began getting glimpses of my future. From what I could make of it, it looked absolutely pathetic. I was hopelessly adrift and, for the first time in four years, I couldn't hide it any longer. Everyone around me seemed to have some sort of a plan—grad school, military service, job interviews. Yet when I tried to think about what I wanted to do after graduation, my mind literally went blank. I didn't like what I could see waiting for me off in the distance.

Despite joining a frat filled with science geeks, so much of my identity over the past few years had been spent trying to find attractive people to hang out with so I could look good. Besides, it was easier for me to care more about others since I firmly believed everyone else was worth more than me. My GPA plummeted because once I got accepted into my frat house, the older members no longer monitored my class activities. When it came to balancing academics and my social life, I was an irresponsible mess. And once it became clear that our house was going to survive, I decided that partying was more important than attending classes. I'd spent the past few years trying to do as little work as possible. I no longer cared about impressing anybody—my parents or my fraternity brothers—so I only bothered attending 20 percent of my classes. I lived for the weekend, for my next beer binge, sexual conquest, or LSD trip. Like it was for a lot of my friends, taking psychedelic drugs had become one of my favorite activities. Strangely, it made me feel more normal, especially when I realized that whenever my friends took a hit of acid, they acted just like me—when I was straight. Suddenly, they saw nothing odd about staring intently at a wood-paneled wall for thirty minutes without blinking.

My father died in his sleep of a heart attack the day after Christmas in 1969. My parents, who had both retired from teaching by then, were living in Santa Monica at the time. When he died, I happened to be visiting Los Angeles—not to see them, but to party with some of my frat buddies and attend the Rose Bowl. Because I never bothered telling anybody in my family how to get hold of me, I didn't learn about his death until two days later. My brother Jim, who lived in the area, told me over the phone when I called to see about bumming a ride with him to our folks' apartment. I didn't cry. I didn't feel much of anything.

My father and I had been drifting apart for several years, ever since that day in high school I grew angry with him over his shoddy treatment of my brother John, when John had turned to him for help when his marriage was crumbling. All my father could do was shout at him, telling him to get his act together. The resentment it caused within me had nothing to do with feelings of empathy for my older brother. My dad's strangely uncaring response convinced me, once and for all, that both my parents were only interested in having poster children. The moment any one of us dared reveal a single human frailty, they wanted nothing to do with us. After that, the two of us rarely spoke. When we did, we couldn't agree on anything. I was fifteen when he had his first stroke. I think my decision to go so far away to school was a relief to him. He had his next stroke when I was twenty, right around the time my GPA was in the final stages of its nosedive. Instead of going through the roof, he heeded his doctors' advice and decided not to let my screwups cause his blood pressure to red-line. Deep down, I now realize he was hoping I could clean up my mess without any interference from him.

After he died, a Presbyterian minister showed up at my mother's apartment and read some prayers to us while we sat around on the sofa in the front room. I didn't want to be at this low-key memorial service for my father. All I could think about was that if the minister didn't stop talking, I was going to miss the date I'd wrangled with a doe-eyed Ukranian girl from Michigan I'd run into at the Rose Bowl.

Everything I'd been dreading came crashing down on me one afternoon the following spring. I suddenly realized I'd actually managed to graduate from college and couldn't postpone my future any longer. Oh, great, I thought, now I'm supposed to go out and get a life. I was living in a run-down house off campus with six buddies I'd met back when I was still allowed to take honors classes. It was the end of April and our lease had just expired. My roommates had already packed up and moved out. The place was empty and barren, except for my filthy room. I sat on my bed with the door shut, trying not to think about what was happening, trying to shut everything out. By the skin of my teeth, I'd managed to get a degree in math and economics. Not that I actually had the diploma, because I'd never bothered attending my graduation ceremony. I'd arrived in Ann Arbor four and a half years before with my head stuffed so full of big plans and ideals I thought it might explode. Everybody around here will know Jerry Newport—that's what I told myself on the morning I first stepped off the Greyhound bus.

Suddenly, the door to my room flew open and a stranger stood there looking at me. I quickly realized he was one of the new tenants, no doubt curious as to why I was still there. I wondered the same thing myself. I jumped up from the bed as though startled from a deep sleep. From the lower part of the house, I could hear the sound of footsteps and boxes being dragged across the floor.

"Oh," he said, looking both surprised and concerned. "I'm gonna be moving in here. You gonna be much longer?"

On an impulse, I quickly started glancing around my room, trying to calculate exactly how many trips up and down the stairs it would take to empty the place of my junk.

"Oh yeah," I replied, trying to feign coolness. "I was wondering when you were gonna get here. . . . I'll be cleared out of here in a few."

Twenty minutes later, I'd thrown all my belongings into the back of our family's old Chevy Impala and started driving. I had absolutely no idea where I was going. But if the gas gauge was correct, I had a quarter of a tank to get there.

TUCSON, ARIZONA
SEPTEMBER 1977

As afternoons went, this one was shaping up to be pretty freaky. I was cowering in a tiny cave, clutching my little boy. Charlie, a former lover who had recently sniffed a bit too much model airplane glue, was hurling large rocks at the cavern's entrance. The racket made by the rocks slamming against the outside of the cave was deafening, the kind of oppressive sound that could send someone like me or Jerry into full meltdown mode. It scares me to think how he would have fared with all that chaotic noise reverberating around him. He often has a rough time with sharp, clattering sounds, while I find it impossible to endure lower-pitched rumbling tones.

I'd met Charlie a few weeks earlier when I picked him up hitchhiking on a nearby highway. Cowering beside me on that afternoon was another scraggly hitchhiker named Running Bear. We'd known each other for three days. Ever since returning from Italy, I'd begun picking up hitchhikers in an effort to meet people, hoping one of them might point me in the direction I needed to go next. I'd moved back into my parents' home. Because they felt a bit guilty over how things had unfolded during my stint with the Children of God, they were trying to be on their best behavior around me. My father, however, didn't hide his feelings about Running Bear.

He looked too much like Charles Manson for him to be comfortable. "I think it's a sexy look," I told my father. "Especially his eyes." But my father called the police on Running Bear when he caught the two of us in the kitchen making fruit smoothies.

After the cops finally left our house, we jumped into my parents' car, drove to a nearby canyon on the outskirts of Tucson, and decided to crash in one of the caves. It was a glorious existence. No one was telling me what to do. The only possessions I brought with me were a sleeping bag, some diapers, a guitar, and a few of Running Bear's artillery handbooks, which he claimed would come in handy when it came time to topple the U.S. government. We'd been there about a month when Charlie showed up in our canyon, high as a kite and heaving rocks at our cave. When I'd met Charlie earlier, he'd filled my head so full of his hippie free-love philosophy that I actually thought he practiced what he preached.

Why, I wondered, after only one sexual encounter, could Charlie be angry with me for spreading my love around? How could anyone be so possessive?

Charlie stood outside our cave and continued heaving football-sized rocks into our home, no doubt hoping one of them would crush me. Because the entrance was so small, everything he threw at us shattered into pieces, then fell to the ground. Running Bear squatted beside me, his usual cool look of aloofness had been replaced by one of sheer terror.

"Calm down," I whispered. "Don't be afraid. That only makes things worse. That's when bad things happen."

I tried to explain how I'd come to enjoy frightening moments like this, the feeling of adrenaline trickling into my bloodstream. This was when the magic happened in life, right when things started turning ugly. Running Bear didn't appear in the mood to listen to my epiphanies. He stared blankly at a tattered book covered with pictures of armored tanks that was lying on the ground. So I sat there on the sandy floor, rocking Steve in my arms, attempting to use my powers of mind control to telepathically convince Charlie to get a grip on his anger and leave us alone. A half hour later, my mind melding worked its magic. Either that, or Charlie ran out of rocks. The last I saw of him, he was stumbling up the canyon, searching for a cave of his own where he could crash.

Before long, Running Bear and I were tangled up in each other on the floor, making love, an exciting departure from the stale, choreographed ritual that sex had become during my marriage to Ace. Steve was napping on my sleeping bag, off in the corner. I didn't care what anybody thought. I truly loved living here. My parents had threatened to take Steve away from me, claiming I was an unfit mother. Normal mothers, the ones who truly cared for their children, lived in houses with shingles on top and grass in the front yard. Even my older brother, Ed, who was unnerved by my decision to become a cave dweller, had begun insisting that my soul had undoubtedly been seized by demons.

I felt sealed off from a world I'd never known, but believed with all my heart had to exist. Like others with autism, I told myself I was locked away in an escape-proof caste system filled with social untouchables just like me. I kept searching for some sort of safety net beneath me, but all I could see was cold, hard-packed dirt. And so I found myself yearning to disappear into nature, to live as far away from society as possible. I wanted to be like that woman in Chapter 12 of the Book of Revelation, the one who flees into the wilderness to escape the evilness unfolding over the earth. Running Bear and I eventually parted ways, and I traveled to Oregon as a favor to one of the hippies we'd lived with in a commune for several months before our split. She needed someone to take her six-year-old son to her brother, who lived at a run-down ranch.

The moment I saw Michael it felt like a floodlight had turned on inside my heart. In a flash, I was in love for the first time in my adult life. Michael, who'd been living on his own since he'd turned sixteen, could play guitar and sing just like Bob Dylan. He was skinny, his nose was big, and he had a mane of dreadlocks hanging from his head that resembled strands of dirty rope. I'd never met anyone like Michael. The first thing I did for him was wash his hair and comb out his dreads. Because I loved him, I wanted people to treat him with more respect. I believed that helping him clean up his act was the first step toward that end.

Our first project together involved building a nest—literally. Using twigs, leaves, branches, ferns, and moss, we fashioned a giant nest in the woods outside Vida, Oregon. We lived like enlightened Neanderthals among the massive ponderosa pines and the occasional mountain lion. The next few months were filled with more bliss than I'd ever believed possible. During the days, I wandered through the forest with Steve, nearly two years old, imagining myself to be a modern-day Eve, explaining everything I knew about nature to him. We'd spend hours staring at slugs, studying their delicate mucus-covered antennas, their mysterious stripes and spots, the pearly, opalescent trails of slime that marked where they'd been. We'd sit beside streams and listen to the plops and gurgles of the flowing water and hear melodies. The wind blowing through the leaves overhead sounded like music.

Sometimes, Michael and I would lie beside each other in our nest of ferns and study each other's faces. Occasionally, I even dared to stare into his eyes, a feat I'd spent much of my life avoiding, resorting to it only when I truly wanted to get something from somebody. As strange as it sounds, my dislike of looking into another person's eyes actually helped heighten my powers of awareness. Most of the time when I spoke to people, my gaze would initially drift to their mouths. I found that people tended to believe they could get away with things because they sensed I was avoiding their eyes. But I learned that the shape of a person's mouth often said just as much as their words. At any given moment, incriminating micro-expressions flashed across people's faces. I was forever on the lookout for smiles, scowls, frowns, or any other subconscious clue that enabled me to read the thoughts behind their words.

My relationship with Michael marked the beginning of another new chapter in my life. For the first time, I felt that I'd found a man who could look past all my weirdness and glimpse into my soul. Like me, Michael had grown so disenchanted with the system that he wanted to live as far away from it as possible. He was also committed to not harming the planet. Even more important, Michael made me feel beautiful. Of course, the honeymoon didn't last forever. We eventually moved to New Mexico to live in a giant teepee I'd stitched together out of new upholstery fabric covered in polyethylene. Together with Michael's sister, we camped in a riverbed, panned for gold, and rock-hounded for semi-precious minerals. Thanks to our food stamps, we ate every type of grain that we could get our hands on. At night, we'd be lulled to sleep by the sound of coyotes laughing and singing in the distance. From day one, I did all of the cooking. Before long, I was the only person willing to do any work around our camp. Michael and his sister would smoke pot, goof on the crazy leaf pattern embroidered on the inside of our teepee, and engage in dopey hippie talk while I gathered firewood, fetched buckets full of water, and racked my brain trying to find new ways to prepare our grains. I actually enjoyed doing the chores and tried to explain how fun they could be if you made a game out of them, but no one was really interested in listening.

I obsessed over death. At night, when the rains came, I worried about what would happen if a flash flood ripped through the area while we lay asleep, eventually realizing that having your lungs fill up with water was a mercifully quick way to die. One afternoon, a warm front moved though area, melting the snowpack that had collected in the mountains above us. The floodwaters came, but they rose so slowly that we had time to clear out of our camp before being swept away. We packed up and eventually ended up back in Oregon, at a hippie enclave where we rented a primitive cabin from a rancher who never seemed interested in collecting our rent money. That spring in central Oregon all it did was rain and sleet. Because our firewood was often too wet to light, the temperature in our tiny cabin always seemed to hover a few degrees above freezing.

Our bodies soon acclimated to the cold. Before long, I'd grown so used to the conditions that I could walk barefoot through the snow. By then, I was six months pregnant with Michael's child. Yet Michael stayed away from me for weeks at a stretch, choosing instead to party away his time with a bunch of hippie guys who lived on the other side of the mountain. His selfishness hurt, but I also felt it a sign of weakness to deny someone pleasure just because of something I wanted. So I kept quiet. I didn't mind being alone. It gave me time to explore my thoughts—to wait for them to present themselves, then I'd pluck them out of my mind and inspect them the way I might examine a moth or a ladybug, turning them over and over in my hand, studying every minute detail. My little boy was the same way. Because he'd never grown up watching television, he could manufacture fun out of just about anything. The two of us would huddle together in our cabin to keep ourselves warm, tell each other simple stories, and sing songs.

One afternoon I fried some falafels out of our ground-up chickpeas and calmly realized that we'd just eaten the last of our food. Instead of panicking, I consciously decided to use this seemingly unpleasant moment as a learning experience. I didn't have any way to get into town through the snow, so Steve and I had no choice but to spend the next few days fasting. The sensation felt exquisite, especially when I noticed how starvation somehow forced my pregnant body's metabolism to slow down. The pain and discomfort gave way to an indescribable sense of bliss.

After my second child, Peter, was born at a healthy, normal weight, we moved into a tiny run-down house in Vida. The previous tenant sold pot and left the basement floor covered in cannabis seeds. That summer, a marijuana jungle had sprouted in the backyard. I was always paranoid that we were on the verge of getting arrested. By this point, Michael's drinking and pot smoking had begun to consume him.

One day, about a week after phoning my parents to see if they could lend me any money, our mailman dropped off a letter containing a $600 check, a portion of a childhood life insurance policy payout. I used the money to purchase a '39 Chevy flatbed truck. Michael replaced the engine. We built a redwood cottage on the back of it, complete with a wood-burning stove and a golden velvet couch, then hit the road selling all sorts of leather goods we'd made at craft shows, swap meets, and art fairs. We had learned how to take a penny's worth of leather, cut it into the shape of a wristband, stamp someone's name into it, put a snap on it, then sell it for a dollar. It was good money, but Michael

eventually couldn't handle the idea that my freehand creations—
such as the two intertwining snakes eating each other (a symbol of
eternity) that I'd put on hair barrettes—would outsell his painstakingly hand-stamped handbags, wallets, and belts. One day he
ordered me to stop making anything else out of leather.

"From here on out, I'm the only one who touches any of this,"
he demanded, pointing to our supply of leather piled on a tiny
workbench. "I don't want you going near it."

His ridiculous directive frustrated me. For the first time in
years, I'd found something I was good at, and I'd truly begun
enjoying the sensation of creating. What's more, we were finally
earning enough money to buy food and bolts of cloth out of which
I stitched clothing for the kids. But I was determined to glimpse
the silver lining inside every storm cloud. That's just the way I
was. And always have been. As dark and dismal as my life often
was, I couldn't shake the feeling that I was blessed and any given
moment—no matter how dark and hopeless it seemed—was just a
test to determine how strong my faith was. So when Michael told
me to stop doing the thing I loved, I told myself that at least he'd
put the brakes on his boozing. He'd stopped being a lazy hippie
and actually wanted to be the family provider. He was trying to
make something of himself. That was the only thing that mattered
to me.

"If that's what you really want me to do," I replied, "then okay."

Money once again began getting tight. But at least I had plenty
of time on my hands to spend playing with my boys and continuing to try to understand everything going on inside my mind. A
hunger had begun to gnaw at me. I yearned to shape my reality
and began to equate the path my life had taken over the years with
the complicated, seemingly unpredictable route that a Super Ball
makes when you toss it against a wall with all your strength. I
wanted not only to predict where that ball would bounce next, but
also to influence its trajectory, to will it into behaving in whatever
way I imagined.

We continued to wander, which seemed like the most natural thing in the world to do. Eventually, because we'd run out of money, I took a job as a cook at a run-down nursing home in Santa Cruz. By the time we moved to an abandoned mushroom farm on a beach north of town, Michael had gotten himself tangled up with another woman. I'd work all day and when I returned home he'd be drinking, smoking pot, and lying in bed with his new lover. One night, I grew so upset over what was happening, I confronted him.

"Michael, we need to talk," I insisted.

"Nothing to talk about," he slurred. "I love her. . . . You know why? Because she's nothing like you. . . . She's cool." He stumbled back to our bed and instantly fell into a deep, drunken sleep. A moment later, I grabbed him by the shoulder and tried to shake him awake. I desperately wanted to talk. When Michael's eyes opened, the look on his face resembled that of a madman. His hands darted upward, grabbed my head, and the next thing I knew he was slamming my forehead against the floor. Even though I knew I should, I didn't feel any pain. All I saw were pretty stars, brilliant cometlike bursts of light. I glimpsed my two boys watching wide-eyed as Mommy's head bounced off the wooden floor like one of those Super Balls she spent so much time pondering. When Michael saw what he'd done, he grabbed Peter, wrapped him in an old flannel shirt, and ran out the door of our camper, disappearing into the chilly, salt air. Deep down, I knew he'd come back the moment he ran out of patience and decided he needed help taking care of Peter, who had just celebrated his first birthday.

The next day I walked to my job, leaving Steve in the capable hands of another mother who had moved into our makeshift camp. It didn't take long before a few of my coworkers confronted me about my bruised face and black eye, which had swollen shut. "You gotta be crazy to put up with that stuff from your old man," a nurse named Rita told me. "Take your kids and get out."

"But I love him and he loves me," I stammered, while Rita rolled her eyes incredulously. "He won't do it again. I just know it."

After work that day, I wandered the halls filled with the catatonic elderly men and women who were being warehoused at the nursing home. Ever since I'd started, I'd always tried to finish my cooking duties early so I could sit with anyone who looked like they wanted to talk or might need company. Even if I couldn't understand their words, I listened to the sounds they'd offer up to me from their throats and managed to feel their emotion and energy. I tried my best to weave together a thread or two of conversation that drifted awkwardly through the disinfectant-laden air.

Most of our charges, however, were so strung out on their medications that all they could do was lie there in bed, staring up listlessly at the dirty acoustic tiles overhead. Sometimes I'd prop up their bony, emaciated bodies and we'd just sit there together in silence, as I listened to their raspy, labored breathing. As nightmarishly empty as their lives had become, I sometimes envied these forgotten octogenarians. Nobody bothered them anymore.

Of all the nursing home residents, Homer was my favorite. And on that afternoon after my beating I found him, as usual, strapped into one of those rickety wooden desk chairs I remembered seeing in elementary schools. "I'm riding my horse," he exclaimed, rocking back and forth, the smile on his leathered face stretched from one wrinkled earlobe to the other. "This ol' mare of mine, she's full of vinegar today. I can barely hold on."

Nobody else seemed to have time for Homer. His brain may have been pumped full of enough tranquilizers to kill one of those imaginary equines he spent his day galloping upon, but something about the twinkle in his eyes convinced me that he was more in control of reality than anyone else at the nursing home—patients or staff.

I pulled up a chair and sat beside him. "How you doing today, Homer?" I asked. He nodded and smiled.

"I'd rather be riding a horse than stay strapped in a chair," he said, then took off at a quick imaginary gallop down the hall, out the front door, and off across the countryside. Without thinking, I shut my eyes and decided to follow him. A moment later, my life was behind me and I was free, holding on to the neck of a gray stallion, the sea air blowing through my hair. Wonderful therapy, horseback riding. After a few minutes, I felt reborn.

"Thanks for letting me come along, Homer," I said. "You keep on riding. I'll see you tomorrow." He flashed me a cowboy grin and continued on down the trail.

Michael returned home with Peter a week later. Not long after that, I quit my job at the nursing home and we moved north to Washington, where we'd heard a radio report that they were hiring apple pickers. Whatever money we earned usually went to buy Michael's booze or pot. One night, he got drunk and threatened to beat me up and disappear with Peter. Up until that moment, whenever he flew into one of his rages, I envisioned myself to be a surfer riding on the wave of his anger, always careful not to get caught inside the tube when his rage inevitably broke. But on that night, I no longer cared what happened. I wasn't going to let him take Peter. Not this time. I telephoned the sheriff. When he arrived, the orchard owner came to my defense, telling the officer how I never got high or drunk and worked harder than anyone else, in between cooking and taking care of my children.

"That one there, he's just one of those no-good stoned hippies," the orchard owner said, pointing to Michael.

The sheriff nodded thoughtfully, then pronounced his verdict. "You'd better clear out, mister," he told Michael. "The children stay with their mother."

A few days later, Peter, Steve, and I were sitting on a DC–10, barreling through the clouds, heading back to Tucson. I'd agreed to give Michael our truck and, once again, telephoned my parents, who had become my last-ditch safety net during my periodic free falls through life. My mother had agreed to send me some airplane tickets.

I was twenty-two years old. I had a sixth-grade education and two kids. Our clothes hung like rags off our bodies. Everything we owned could fit into a single bag. Yet I couldn't have been happier. For the first time in my life, despite what anyone else said or thought, I understood that I wasn't some stupid, spaced-out moron. Deep in my heart, I knew I was capable of thinking profound thoughts, of creating beautiful things.

When I arrived in Arizona, I planned to take classes at the university, to study music and learn everything I could about composition, theory, and performance. My mother had agreed to look after the boys while I was away at school. I thought back on the past seven years, took a deep breath, and went to work constructing a little black box inside my head to store all the moments I'd just lived through since being shipped off to the Children of God. Beside me, Peter and Steve had their faces pressed against the porthole-like window of the jet. The scorched brown earth of Arizona rolled out beneath us like a dirty carpet. Before long, I could feel the drag of the landing gear being lowered beneath the belly of our plane. I went back to stuffing my past into the box. By the time we landed and pulled up beside the terminal, everything was packed away inside my head. I shut the lid, sealed it tightly, gathered up my boys, and stepped off the jet into the blistering Arizona heat, into what I hoped would be the first page of a new chapter in my life.

CHAPTER SIX

I wasn't in the best of moods on that evening my telephone rang. I'd spent another long, frustrating day racing through Los Angeles traffic, delivering blueprints to architects' offices as part of my latest dead-end job as a courier. At the moment, I was attempting to construct a Willy the Whale costume out of chicken wire and papier-mâché. I decided Willy would be my perfect guise for the upcoming Halloween costume party I'd organized for my autism support group. By then, I'd watched *Free Willy* six times. I liked the way Willy made friends with the boy in the movie. And I loved the scene where the boy first touched Willy, who desperately yearned to be touched but was just as frightened of physical contact as I was when I was a boy. (As much as I hated to admit it, I sometimes felt like Willy because of all the extra weight I'd packed on since college.)

Ever since my graduation, two and a half decades earlier, I'd not only packed on the pounds, I'd drifted from one failed vocation to the next—pot dealer, horse-race betting fanatic, taxi driver, Goodwill bell ringer, bookstore cashier, elementary school librarian, and probably a half dozen other jobs I've purged from my memory. I was as lost and hopelessly adrift as a person could be and still function. Nevertheless, there were moments when I glanced out over the horizon and caught glimpses of land, when I regained my bearings. And on two occasions, those moments came after I watched a movie. As strange as it sounds, Hollywood helped give me a better understanding of who I was.

The second time that happened was when I watched *Free Willy,* which would explain why I went to the trouble of constructing a whale costume. But the first time a movie touched me in a place that I never knew existed was when I bought a ticket to see *Rain Man.* One hundred and thirty-three minutes later, I was never the same again. That was back on a cool Sunday in the autumn of 1989. I arrived at the theater just before the matinee started, grabbed a soda and a hot dog, then plopped myself down in the second-row seat, not quite sure what to expect. Yet the moment I saw Raymond Babbitt shuffling across the screen, I couldn't take my eyes off of him. Never in my life had I so identified with a movie character. Why on earth would I? After all, nobody in any movie I'd ever watched was remotely like me. And even though I knew Raymond was fictional, I couldn't help thinking I was looking at a faint shadow of myself. All of Raymond's kooky traits felt so familiar. But the real kicker came when a doctor asked Raymond's brother, Charlie, played by Tom Cruise, "Can he multiply?"

I couldn't believe what I was hearing, so I just sat there with my mouth open, fighting the urge to scream "That's just like me! That's just like—" Suddenly, I forgot I was sitting in a movie theater. No sooner had Raymond been asked to multiply two six-digit numbers than I shouted out the answer, a split second before Raymond could open his mouth.

"Shhhhhhhh," I heard someone whisper behind me.

"Shut up, will ya?" someone else yelled.

I slunk down in my seat, feeling as though I'd just found my long-lost brother. Something about him reminded me of that so-called idiot savant my frat brothers had compared me to. After all these years, I realized that maybe there was a bit of truth to what they had said. And when the movie finally ended, I practically skipped out of the darkened theater, out into the late afternoon sunlight. When I spotted the movie poster in the lobby, I rushed over to it and for some reason felt compelled to gently touch the top of Raymond's head with the tips of my fingers. Then I just stood there for what seemed like hours.

"It's too bad they had to put you back in that institution, Raymond," I heard myself whisper. "It sure seems like there should have been some way to keep you out."

The two attendants behind the snack bar were staring at me when I finally turned to leave and begin my walk back home. I'd covered less than a block when I got one of those ideas that I immediately sensed had the potential to forever change my life. Maybe, I thought, if I learn more about Raymond, I'll learn more about me. I knew Raymond Babbitt was an autistic savant. I identified with that part of him. Yet judging from what little I knew about the disorder, I didn't feel autistic. I told myself I was too in control of my own life. But there was no denying that the two of us had much in common. His social naïveté made me feel like I was staring into a mirror—the way he stopped in the middle of that crosswalk after the signal read Don't Walk; the way he knew all the intro songs and slogans for my three favorite TV shows—*The People's Court, Jeopardy,* and *Wheel of Fortune*—nearly knocked me out of my seat; his meltdown over the ringing smoke detector; how he loved to watch socks spin around in the dryer at the Laundromat; his penchant for mathematics.

After the movie, I phoned my middle brother, Jim, a Hollywood art director. He suggested that I go to the library and find out who the technical consultants for the movie were. It didn't take long before I tracked down the name of the world-renowned San Diego psychologist Dr. Bernard Rimland, whose 1964 classic book, *Infantile Autism,* helped debunk the commonly held theory that autism resulted from having a cold, uncaring mother. I wrote Dr. Rimland a letter and over the course of several pages, I told this complete stranger all about my frustrating, empty life. A couple of weeks later, he wrote back informing me that it sounded as if I exhibited all the symptoms of someone with autism or something close to it. He urged me to learn everything I could about this disorder, but cautioned me against reading too many autobiographies penned by autistics, especially while I was still unsure if I was actually autistic.

"It might confuse you about your own life," he wrote, explaining that each autistic person is so unique that one story can't even begin to encapsulate another's experience. I didn't know it at the time, but *Rain Man* was also inspiring a lot of autism wannabes, people looking for an exotic excuse to be weird and get government assistance while doing it. For all I knew, I could be another one of those poseurs. Nevertheless, for the next few months, I camped out in the aisles of the Santa Monica Public Library, devouring everything I could locate on the subject. But the more I read, the less autistic I felt. Over time, I began to see myself as the man without a diagnosis.

Then one day I stumbled upon a copy of Temple Grandin's book *Emergence: Labeled Autistic,* and something clicked inside me. Here was a true savant, someone who had managed to harness her unique skills to become a university professor and the world's leading expert in the design of slaughterhouses. I soon learned that she had a form of autism known as Asperger's syndrome, which I quickly began to view as "autism lite." What truly set those with Asperger's apart was their chronic inability to handle social relationships. By the time I'd finished Temple's book, I realized there were other people out there just like me. I'd found a kindred spirit. God only knew how many others were out there just like her. Just like me?

It took me years to get up enough nerve to finally answer that question. By the fall of 1989, I'd joined a local running club to train for the Los Angeles marathon. Running track had been the only thing that had consistently helped calm me down and kept me focused in high school. Two decades later, when I learned about the city's twenty-six-mile race, I became hooked on running again and began looking forward to the weekly training runs. At the end of each Saturday morning's run, the club gathered in a local elementary school cafeteria and we listened as members stood up and gave motivational speeches. I'd made the mistake of telling the club founder, Bob Scott, about my exploration of autism and how running had helped give me a sense of control over my life. One Saturday, when our designated speaker didn't show up, Bob asked if I wouldn't mind sharing my story with the group.

"Why not?" I shrugged. And for the next half hour I stood there on the edge of the stage, alone, in front of nearly two hundred people, telling them about the journey I'd secretly been taking over the past year. Despite my often stammering, rambling monotone, nobody in the room stirred. On account of all the running I'd done before speaking, my nerves weren't a problem. So all I did was open my mouth and I felt this sensation, almost like I had this conveyor belt that stretched from my heart to my lips—the words just dropped onto it and were pulled effortlessly out of my chest, out to the awaiting ears of my fellow would-be marathoners. That moment marked a turning point in my life.

"You know, ever since seeing *Rain Man,* I've wondered whether autism and I had anything in common," I stammered. "But that's not what I want to talk about. I just want to share with you how being a runner and a volunteer with this group has reminded me of something I'd forgotten. That those few things that have helped me gain contact with the outside world are the same things which tend to lift up groups of people, as opposed to individuals. What all of you have helped me learn during these past two seasons spent running with you is much more important than answering the question of whether or not I'm autistic. You've reminded me that if one's life is to mean anything, it can only occur when we set out to try to elevate others—only then do we end up elevating ourselves. For those of us here, it happens when we realize that our individual times in the coming marathon aren't important. What is important is that we all finish the race as a family, as a running community."

Up until that day, I rarely realized the impact of what I'd said—both on me or others—until long after I'd uttered it. It was a neurological shortcoming that had wreaked unimaginable havoc in my life. But that wasn't the case as I stood up there and finally allowed my heart to speak for me. Every single person in that auditorium had not only helped me prepare for a twenty-six-mile race, but had also assisted me in a personal journey to understand who Jerry Newport was. And I'd tried to do likewise. As corny as it sounds, I had arrived. I had finally grown from a perpetually insecure, ego-driven lost soul into somebody who found happiness in doing things he believed in for the greater good of those around him. My wealth, I knew for the first time in my life, would never come from money, but from a source far more important and lasting: my relationships with the people around me.

When I finished speaking, people started clapping, the kind of clapping where you can't help but jump up on your feet and begin slapping your hands together to make as much noise as possible. A few people even whistled. The club's founder walked up on stage and hugged me.

"What you're doing could probably help some other people," a young woman in yellow sweatpants told me as the crowd filed out of the cafeteria. "But you're never going to find out what sort of an impact you could have unless you contact some autistic organization. I'm sure there must be some in Los Angeles."

She was right, of course. Despite all my searching, I'd never quite struck up the courage to contact the Autism Society of Los Angeles. This was due to one simple, yet pathetic reason: I was deathly afraid they'd turn me away. After finally convincing myself that I'd stumbled upon a way to define myself, I was terrified at the

possibility of being cast back out into a world where I'd never fit
in. Nevertheless, since so many of my fellow runners had been kind
enough to spend a half hour of their time listening to my story, I
felt obligated to suck it up and attend the group's next meeting.

Much to my relief, they welcomed me. And by the spring of
1992, I parlayed all the skills I'd gleaned from my days spent in
the San Diego taxi driver's union in the mid-1980s and got myself
elected to the organization's board of directors. The notion of my
rubbing shoulders with some of the most respected names in the
autism world never ceased to make me smile. It also emboldened
me, got me thinking about other ways I might be able to put my
life experiences to better use.

Together with my first autistic friend and jogging buddy,
Jonathan Mitchell, I began kicking ideas around. Eventually, we
came up with a truly novel gem: why not create a support group
solely for and run entirely by adult autistics? I couldn't understand why no one had ever attempted anything like it. Up until
then, it seemed that when we adults with autism got together to
talk about our lives, we always had our hands held by well-intentioned parents and caregivers. The experience was not only un-
intentionally demeaning, it was debilitating. The more I thought
about it, the more I realized that our community seemed to know
much more about the first twenty years of an autistic person's life
than it did about the *rest* of that life. And that just seemed unac-
ceptable to me.

"It would just be nice to have a place where we didn't have
to apologize for what we are," said Jonathan, who had received
his diagnosis when he was a kid, then went on to receive a degree
in psychology from UCLA. I couldn't have agreed more and felt
excited to help try to create a sort of virtual safety zone for the
adults who had finally admitted we were too old to be cured and
desperately yearned for a break from our all-too-often supervised
lifestyles.

Three months later, at the tail end of a conference on adult autism issues held in Long Beach, California, fourteen of us met in the corner of the auditorium. The event's moderator, a part-time stand-up comedian who happened to be the older brother of an autistic adult, presided over the group. We were a diverse lot, which included a grandmother, a couch potato, a mother of two, and a long-distance runner on the Long Beach City College track team. Over the next hour, we hashed out exactly what each of us wanted to get from a group like this. I commandeered a blackboard and scribbled down everyone's wish list—things like information on autism, job leads, social opportunities, comfort, and recreational options. When it became evident that we were actually going to meet again, I drew a makeshift map of LA on the board and began putting X's where everyone lived. Since a majority of the group lived near Culver City, we decided to hold our next gathering a month later at the home of a woman who lived in the area. And when it became apparent that our first meeting was over, I was the last man left sitting. On the way out, somebody dumped the sign-up sheet in my lap.

"Congratulations," chuckled our moderator. "Looks like you're the leader."

"Leader by default," I laughed.

By the end of the summer of 1993, we came up with a name for our truly unorthodox group—AGUA, which stood for Adults Gathering United Autistic. The acronym for our organization—AGUA—means water in Spanish. Many of us joked that autism was really our first language and English our second. It only seemed natural that anyone who wanted to know about our group would have to learn at least one word in another language. By then, our membership swelled to a whopping twenty-four people. With each meeting we held, our members grew more relaxed with one another. Dean was a perfect example. The first time he showed up, he wandered about the room talking to himself about his various interests, such as the space program or gardening. But over time, he began to feel comfortable enough to share his hobbies with anyone willing to converse with him.

Before long, the group had become much more male than female, which proved disappointing to a number of the guys who would attend one meeting desperately looking for a mate, then never return. It always made me sad that they didn't stick around just to have some friends. They would have certainly discovered plenty of them. We had so many characters in our midst, there was never a dull moment. Glenn was a perfect example. Incredibly high functioning and addicted to structure, he worked as an accountant, and each day he followed the most rigid, activity-packed schedule imaginable, which included everything from clarinet lessons to self-defense classes. Glenn drove, too, but it was difficult for him to deviate from the menu of roads he knew. AGUA helped loosen him up just a bit, allowing him to become a tad more tolerant of situations and moments that weren't part of his schedule.

The more our group met, the more I allowed myself to believe that I'd finally done something for all the right reasons—and not just because it was going to make me look good. I was also having the time of my life, getting to know others who had been through most of the same battles as I had. Within a short time, we'd become a close-knit band of brothers and sisters.

But it wasn't all good times. One of our early members eventually had to be asked to leave. The notion that he needed support beyond what we could provide proved to be a sad and frustrating situation for all of us. I'll never forget the meeting when our steering committee came to its decision. We were all feeling pretty glum—that is, until one of our members said with absolute seriousness: "You know, even we have standards."

It wasn't long after that, on a humid evening in September 1993, when the telephone in my apartment rang. I was clumsily attempting to piece together my whale costume for our AGUA Halloween party. I picked up the phone and heard a woman's voice on the other end of the line.

"Hello," she said breathlessly. "My name is Mary Meinel. . . ."

She sounded frantic, lost in a world of confusion and hurt. Her voice had this whiny, nasal drone to it and, before I knew what was happening, she launched into a lengthy monologue about how messed up her life had become. Someone had told her about AGUA and she wanted to attend a meeting. Yet there was also an intriguing, lush quality to her voice, something I rarely heard from other autistic women. It seemed strained, too, as if part of her was as tired of living as I often felt, like she was hanging on to this world by a thin, frayed thread. I definitely could relate—that was, if I'd wanted to. The thing was, I didn't want to. All I really wanted to do was hang up the phone and get back to work on my ridiculous-looking whale costume.

"Our Halloween party is in Long Beach," I told her. "Why don't you try to come?"

She promised she would. I gave her directions to the party, then hung up and quickly forgot all about Mary Meinel.

Less than a month later, Mary wandered out of a bathroom at the AGUA Halloween party, wearing a lavender lace dress and a powder-white wig pulled down over her shaved head. I had no earthly idea who she was, but she looked gorgeous, electric, and somewhat annoyed. I wondered if my incessant pounding on the bathroom door—due to my nearly bursting bladder—might have had something to do with the expression on her face.

"Hi, I'm Jerry Newport," I said.

"Hello, Jerry Newport," she replied. "I'm Mary Meinel."

She seemed nice enough—especially her eyes. Not that I'd really ever spent much time looking at the eyes of other people, but hers felt so alive that I couldn't help myself. Although I didn't see Mary again for another hour, I couldn't help hearing her. Her excited voice thundered through the party like the explosion from a Howitzer. Several of our more timid, sound-sensitive members were so put off by her loudness that they retreated into the kitchen. I watched them cowering in the corner in bewilderment. A few felt compelled to wander over to me and sheepishly complain about her. All I could do was nod sympathetically.

"Hey, at least she's enjoying herself," I replied, pleased that we'd finally attracted someone with a bit of energy to the group. After all, it was far easier to deal with someone with excess energy than to spend all your time attempting to jump-start individuals. Which was what I often ended up doing at our gatherings with several of our members, who could actually sit in a meeting for two hours and never utter a single word.

Naturally, Mary was a hit with a few of the more outgoing guys in the group. By the time I got around to speaking to her again, she was standing in a corner of the room as they showered her with attention. Instead of basking in it—like several of the females in AGUA would have done—she laughed it off and peppered her admirers with a barrage of questions. Did they have any hobbies? Did they ever feel lonely? What was it that made them happiest in life? I'd never seen or heard anything like it. She was truly interested in everything about them. Whenever they'd talk, her eyes seemed to ignite and crackle with life.

So, with my half-finished whale costume dangling off me like some narcoleptic Siamese twin, I walked over to her. Jonathan Mitchell saw me approaching and happily began gushing about my number-crunching abilities. All I could do was take a deep breath and sigh. Here we go again. Over these past few years, I'd finally begun to embrace my savantism. Instead of feeling angry or ashamed about it, I ... well, I suppose I learned to tolerate it a bit better.

"You're a savant." She laughed. "I am too. I paint and make music."

"They say that nearly twenty percent of us Aspies are savants," I replied. Mary clapped her hands together and laughed. I looked around the room, not quite sure what to say next. Story of my life.

"So, do your trick," she commanded me, then giggled.

I looked over at Jonathan. He was clearly waiting for my performance. I took another deep breath and asked Mary, "When were you born?"

She told me and my brain went into autopilot, grinding order out of the variables she'd just handed me. She looked amused when I told her what day of the week she was born on.

Afterward, we chatted for a few moments. I complimented her on what a nice Mozart she made. She told me she really liked my Willy. "It's okay you didn't finish it," she said reassuringly. "I can see where you were going with it. You're quite an artist."

I'd been called plenty of things in my life, but no one had ever referred to me as an artist. All I could do was laugh and stare down at the hardwood floor. At that moment, I didn't want to look at her. I just wanted to hold the concept of her in my mind. She seemed nice. That's what I thought. She seemed like the kind of person we needed in AGUA, the kind of person I wouldn't mind having for a friend.

"I'll see you later," I stammered. Then my bedraggled whale costume and I swam away to the kitchen to get a soda.

HOLLYWOOD, CALIFORNIA
SEPTEMBER 1993

The evening I finally got around to telephoning this Jerry Newport character I'd been hearing so much about definitely wasn't one of my best. I'd been through a rough couple of decades. I'd endured more mental breakdowns than I could count. But in between all the sadness and madness, I worked to harness my finely tuned ear to become a concert piano tuner in Los Angeles and New York. Of course, that promising career went up in smoke a few years back, partially due to so many pianos being replaced by synthesizers, and I'd been living on welfare, handouts from my folks, and the occasional odd job ever since.

A few months before I first dialed Jerry's number, I'd shaved my head with a disposable razor and decided to finally act on one of my biggest fantasies—I was going to become a Hollywood extra. Not long afterward, I showed up at a cattle-call audition for a new TV series, *Star Trek: Deep Space Nine*. They needed extras and the minute one of the casting directors spotted me, he chuckled. "Looks like you're ready to play an alien."

When I heard that, all I could do was laugh. "I've been an alien my entire life," I replied.

One week later, I found myself sitting in a chair at the Paramount Studios in Hollywood while a makeup specialist covered me in blue body paint. I'd been tapped to play a hairless, indigo-tinted creature from the planet Bole. Talk about perfect casting. From a psychological standpoint, the two of us could have been twins. She was sneaky, aloof, quiet, and perpetually soaking up everything that went on around her like a sponge. The work was hardly steady, barely enough to support me. But I loved going to the set and spending four hours undergoing the star treatment from the hair and makeup personnel. I may have been only an extra, but before long my strange blue mug even appeared on *Star Trek* trading cards.

All that, however, wasn't enough to prevent me from once again ascending Mount Psycho and contemplate hurling myself off. One afternoon, following a day spent on the *Star Trek* set, I began to seriously ponder shooting a former lover who had just dumped me for another woman. Even though our relationship had recently bit the dust, he could often be found standing beneath my apartment window, hurling insults up at me. Which was one of the reasons why I'd purchased an old Beretta pistol at a nearby pawnshop a few days earlier. Deep down, I truly never intended on pulling the trigger. The gun was merely a version of a scarecrow. But one afternoon, it dawned on me what I'd done: I'd actually purchased a real pistol. And that terrified me. My god, I thought, look how far I've sunk! I picked up the telephone and called the psychiatric ward at USC University Hospital, then tried to admit myself.

It didn't work. The people I spoke with weren't convinced I was dangerous or crazy enough to warrant a stay in their psych wards. I hung up the phone and flopped down beside my kitchen table, wondering what I should do next. A few minutes later, I felt a bizarre urge to telephone my brother David, a Lutheran minister in Dallas, to whom I hadn't spoken in nearly two decades. A few minutes later, after getting his number from directory information, I heard his voice drifting out of my phone.

"David," I said, staring at the Beretta, "it's me, Mary. Your sister."

"Hello, Mary," he said patiently, sounding as though he truly regretted answering the phone. No doubt my parents had kept him up to speed on my exploits over the years.

"How have you been?" he asked.

"Not good," I told him. "I ... I think I'm on the verge of a nervous breakdown."

Even though I was more than a couple thousand miles away from him, I could hear David take a deep, slow breath, then let out a weary sigh. He definitely didn't sound to be in a talkative mood. Not that I could blame him. Why on earth would he want to speak with me? He'd run out of patience for me long before I crashed and burned in junior high.

"Mary," he said after a long pause. "I think you need to call the National Autism Society. I think they can help you."

"Your son's autistic, isn't he?" I asked, attempting to jump-start a conversation. "That's what Mom told me."

"I think you need to call them, Mary," he said. Then he gave me the number, wished me good luck, and quickly hung up the phone.

Autism? I thought to myself. He thinks I'm autistic? I stood there in the kitchen, trying to wrap my mind around the concept. It wasn't as though I'd never pondered the possibility. Months before, while struggling through yet another period where I couldn't communicate with anyone, where dredging up the appropriate words to fit my thoughts seemed like an impossible task, I did some research at the library and stumbled upon a fact that nearly knocked me over: people with autism are often plagued with the exact same inability to express themselves. The next morning I dialed the phone number my brother had given me and eventually reached a woman who patiently listened to my story.

"You know who you should call?" she replied. "His name is Jerry Newport. He recently started up this group that meets once a month, not far from where you live. I think you'd find him interesting."

"Jerry Newport," I said. "Why not? You have his number?"

On the table beside my pistol sat a pastel crayon. I grabbed it and flipped over an unpaid gas bill.

"You ready?" she asked.

"Sure," I told her. "I'm ready."

This Jerry Newport character definitely sounded a bit cranky when I finally got him on the phone. Over the past few weeks, I'd left a handful of messages for him, but he never bothered to call me back. Story of my life: I hit rock bottom, reached out to someone for help, and ended up getting the cold shoulder. Nevertheless, something about the kooky, endearing outgoing message he left on his answering machine intrigued me every time I called it: "You've reached the home of Jerry Newport and the Fantastic Four—Pagliacci, Isadora Duncan, Caruso, and Cockatiel Dundee. Nobody's home. Leave a message."

One evening in September, I told myself I'd dial his number one last time. A few rings later, he picked up the phone.

"Hello!" he yelled into the receiver, sounding like some crabby thug from Brooklyn. His voice was flat, monotone, loud, and possessed an unmistakably annoyed inflection. Yet buried within all that noise, my sensitive ears detected something else, a faint sort of compassion, raw honesty, and hurt that I'd rarely heard before. It was as though I'd stumbled upon a strange new instrument but couldn't quite make sense of the notes it produced. Nevertheless, the moment Jerry picked up the receiver, I pounced, quickly launching into a breathless, fast-paced account of who I was and why I was calling. Unfortunately, he didn't sound interested in anything I felt compelled to say.

"Are you busy?" I asked. "You want me to call back?"

"No," he stammered, explaining that he was in the middle of trying to construct a whale costume for the Halloween party his organization was throwing in three weeks. "I'm not having much luck," he griped. "It sure doesn't look like any whale I've ever seen."

We spoke for several minutes as I tried to pluck whatever information I could from him about his autism group. Every so often, our conversation got severed whenever the wires in the back of my decrepit, antiquated telephone fell out. I was so broke that I couldn't afford to get a new one.

"What's wrong with your phone?" Jerry loudly demanded to know each time I reconnected the wires. "Why don't you get that fixed?" The fact that someone was getting annoyed over something I'd done hardly fazed me. After a lifetime spent ticking people off, I'd long ago grown used to receiving that sort of reaction. Besides, I was too excited over the realization that I may have finally found a group of outcasts with whom I could identify. And the longer I remained on the phone with this foul-tempered stranger, I wondered why on earth I'd never explored the idea that I might have something in common with autistics. Suddenly, I remembered my first-grade teacher, the one who had been perplexed over why I seemed to be incapable of hearing what was being said in class. At a parent-teacher conference, she dropped hints that I might be autistic, an idea my mother quickly dismissed. Not that my mother had anything against autistics. One of our neighbor's daughters, who spent most of her time memorizing cookbooks, had been diagnosed as one.

"She's intelligent in a secret way that not many people can understand," my mother once told me. "She just can't express it in a normal way."

The squawking of Jerry's birds in my receiver pulled me back into the present. It sounded like he lived in a pet shop. "I've got two cockatiels—Ricky and Lucy," I told him excitedly.

"I've got four," he replied, sounding increasingly anxious to terminate our conversation. "You know, I really need to get back to my costume."

As rude as I felt he was being toward me, I found myself enamored with the idea of this man I'd never met, scurrying around alone in his apartment, surrounded by his birds, trying to construct a giant whale suit. It represented the ultimate creative act.

"Well, good-bye," I said

"Yeah ... good-bye," he said, slamming the phone down.

Before Jerry's costume party, I hit a handful of thrift stores in Hollywood and began assembling the perfect costume. I decided to usurp the identity of Nannerl Mozart, Wolfgang's brilliant but forgotten older sister. A musical prodigy whose skills on the piano originally received top billing over those of her brother, she had, with her brother, traveled for years throughout the capitals of Europe playing duets for the day's royalty. By the time Nannerl turned sixteen, her father was more interested in marrying her off than in listening to her brilliant compositions. After her mother died, she spent most of her time doing housework. Despite Wolfgang's urging, she rarely touched the keys of a piano or harpsichord again. Eventually, her father married her off to a widowed magistrate with three kids. When he died, she supported herself by giving piano lessons in Salzburg, Austria. Whenever I thought about Nannerl, I couldn't help experiencing a twinge of kinship and sadness, wondering what musical gifts she might have gone on to create if only given the chance.

Four weeks after my somewhat forgettable conversation with Jerry Newport, I shoved my powder-white wig and my five-dollar lavender lace dress into a backpack, pulled on my bicycle shorts, and climbed onto my ten-speed. Over the next few hours, I pedaled nearly forty miles through Los Angeles traffic, all the way to Long Beach, to the home of the mother of an autistic man, where the AGUA costume party was being held. Upon arriving, I disappeared into the bathroom, sponged off my glaze of sweat, and slipped into my costume. I'm not exactly sure when the banging on the door started, but judging from the intensity of it, somebody definitely needed to use the facilities.

"Just a minute!" I shouted, making a few last-minute adjustments to my wig. "I'll be right out!"

Less than a minute later, the pounding resumed. "Come on!" a voice yelled. "You're keeping people waiting!"

When I finally opened the door, I spotted a bear of a man doing a little jig, holding his crotch. "I thought I was going to wet my pants out here," he explained, still sounding a bit peeved. I was preparing to tell him how one can utilize the muscles in one's pelvic region to prevent incontinence, but decided to introduce myself instead.

"Hi, I'm Mary Meinel," I said. "You must be Jerry Newport."

"Hi," he replied, still doing his cute I-don't-want-to-pee-in-my-pants shuffle. "I've really got to use the bathroom." He disappeared into the restroom and slammed the door shut. I didn't give the incident a second thought. Instead, I gazed out over the small group of people who'd turned out for the party. All it took was a glance and I immediately knew. Nearly everyone in the room stood around looking awkward in a way I knew I'd felt a million times before. At the same time, they also appeared happy to be there, yet unsure why.

A warm feeling rose up inside my chest. I knew I'd finally found a group of hopeless misfits exactly like me. I was so excited that I wanted to run into the middle of the room and begin dancing with joy. I began introducing myself to everybody. And before I knew it, I was immersed in a conversation with an extremely intelligent thirty-something-year-old character, named Robert Green. He wore a black-and-white prison uniform. A collection of old, battered license plates dangled from his shirt and pants. Robert quickly proved himself to be an awful bigot, but there was something so endearingly honest about him that I couldn't help but like him.

"I've never been on a single date in my life," he confessed. "Women don't like me. They won't talk to me."

"Well, I like you," I replied. "And I'm talking to you. We're having a genuine conversation."

Tears began to seep out of Robert's eyes. "I've always felt ugly," he exclaimed. "All my life, I've always felt ugly."

"You're definitely not ugly," I assured him. He looked as though he almost believed me. And then because of our kindred love of science, we began talking about how a beam of light bends and slows down when it passes through various translucent materials. All at once, it hit me that I was engaged in the kind of conversation I could never have with standard-issue humans. I looked around the room. Surrounding me were a sea of people, all locked away in the same sort of prison I'd been confined to my whole life. Each of them was stuck inside a private universe so exotic and complex that attempting to convey it to anyone dwelling in the outside world was an exercise in futility, a recipe for extreme frustration. The only difference between their prison and mine was that the warden granted me more choices, more interests that I could use as bait to communicate with people. It was as though nearly everyone at this costume party received only a couple of channels, while I somehow got satellite TV. I could feel their isolation, and it forced a wave of profound sadness to sweep over me.

Judging by the stares I was getting from the men, I quickly got the feeling that women were something of a rarity at these AGUA shindigs. It didn't take long for Jonathan Mitchell and someone else, who was so shy I never quite heard his name, to wander over and join Robert and me.

"Hey, Mary," Jonathan said, when he spotted a half-finished, bedraggled whale costume lumbering toward us. "Have you met Jerry? He's one of those math geniuses. Aren't you, Jerry?"

"Yes, we met a few minutes ago," I replied. "Jerry was having bladder problems."

Jerry flashed a bashful smile and stared down at the floor. When he wasn't shouting or being cranky, he looked downright sweet—or at least pleasantly less volatile.

"Do your thing for her, Jerry," pleaded another AGUA member, standing beside us. "Do your birthday trick for Mary."

Which is exactly what he did. I told him the date of my birth and a split second later he regurgitated the day of the week it fell on. I had no idea if he was right because I'd never bothered learning which day I'd entered this world on. So much of my life had been spent wishing I'd never been born in the first place. What I did know is that Jerry had the most peculiar look on his face when he performed for me—a peculiar blend of expressions that fluctuated somewhere between sadness, resignation, and anger. I'd never seen anything quite like it.

By this point in the night, he was wearing his whale costume— if you could call it that. It was easily the saddest-looking creation I'd ever seen. The longer I stared at it, the more closely it resembled the decomposing carcass of a whale, washed up on some beach. Jerry hadn't gotten around to finishing it, so it consisted of an exposed chicken-wire frame with a bit of papier-mâché skin hanging off it. Yet despite its ridiculous appearance, there was a certain genius to it. Jerry had managed to capture the distinct shape of a leviathan in the most brilliantly cartoonish manner imaginable.

"I really love your whale costume," I told him, trying to sound earnest. "It's crude but truly wonderful."

"Yeah, well, it still has a ways to go," Jerry said. Our eyes met for a few awkward seconds before each of us looked away, trying to make sense out of what we'd both glimpsed in each other's faces. If I wasn't mistaken, for a fleeting instant something resembling a grin danced across Jerry's face. Try as I might, outside of my sons, I couldn't remember the last time I'd caused such a reaction in another human. A moment later, Jerry turned and lumbered away. So I stood there, stroking the locks of my white wig, watching him and his half-finished whale disappear into the kitchen.

What on earth was that? I asked myself. More than a decade later, I'm still trying to figure out the answer to that question.

CHAPTER SEVEN

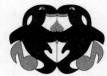Four weeks after we first set eyes on each other, a much less excitable Mary showed up at our next AGUA meeting. This time, instead of dominating the gathering with her manic energy and booming voice, she doted on anyone in attendance who looked as though they were having a tough time venturing outside of their cerebral shell. She seemed to be going out of her way to let people know that she thought they were special. Never before had I seen a woman do anything so sexy. Just the thought of it caused a peculiar mix of emotions to flood through my body.

I suppose that's when the caring began.

The next day, she telephoned and said something to me I'd never heard before. "It would be nice," she suggested, "to spend some time together."

A date? I was being asked out on a date by a woman who I was actually interested in. "How about the racetrack?" I blurted out.

Since neither of us owned a car, Mary thought the zoo would make a better destination. A week later, I showed up at her apartment with dribbles of ketchup smeared all over the front of my

T-shirt. I know she noticed the mess, but she never said anything about it as we rumbled up Hollywood Boulevard on the city bus. Along the way, I read billboards backward and did all sorts of number tricks with the license plates of cars we passed. I wasn't showing off—that was just my only way of calming my nerves.

"Sorry for being so silly," I apologized once I realized what I was doing.

"Don't say you're sorry," Mary told me. "Keep it coming. I think it's great."

We ended up spending a couple of hours wandering around the zoo. As usual, I was constantly counting my steps, trying to measure the distance from one spot to the next. But I was also truly enjoying the animals. And it felt so calming, so right and natural finally to be with someone who saw the world in much the same way I did. From the corner of my eye, I peeked at Mary watching the animals and it made my heart race. Every time she glimpsed another resident of the zoo, her face lit up like a neon sign doused in gasoline—just like mine. Strange, after all these years of being alone, I'd long ago stopped imagining a woman like Mary could ever exist.

By the time we left the zoo and were standing around waiting to catch the bus back to Mary's apartment, tears had pooled in my eyes. I stood there watching her through the salty liquid, and the image was so wonderfully distorted that I pretended I was look-ing through a stained glass window. I could have sworn I heard the voice of God (he actually sounded just like Charlton Heston) telling me: "Here's your reward, Jerry. . . . Here's the gift you've earned for the rotten life I've made you endure."

Mary and I tried taking things slowly, but on Christmas night, two weeks after our first kiss, we made love. We were at my apartment and Mary walked back into my bedroom, turned off the lights, took off her clothes, and lay down on my dirty bed.

"Merry Christmas," she whispered.

Although I didn't have a fraction of the experience that she'd racked up in these matters, she was patient with me, which put me at ease in a way I'd never been before with a woman. And when it was all over and we were lying there in my apartment, I realized something that would have struck me as heretical several years before. I realized that for once in my life, sex no longer mattered to me. All at once it hit me that I'd wasted far too much time in life cooking up this strange testosterone-tinged fantasy of the perfect sexual playmate—someone I could bed, then parade around in front of the world to prove what a man I'd become.

To hell with sex, I told myself. All I want now is a friend.

Thank God, Mary couldn't hear my thoughts because I considered her to be an incredibly sexy creature. Her beautiful, magically symmetrical face crackled with electricity whenever she smiled, which was constantly. Because of all the bicycle riding she did, she was also in terrific shape, and I longed for those moments when she'd drape those warm, muscular legs over mine and talk to me in her sensual voice. Up until the moment that thought trickled through my brain, I had no appreciation of what it meant to have a woman as a real partner in life. Mary changed all that. We could talk about anything. We didn't feel nervous around each other. Nothing seemed to bother us about each other.

I soon began to revel in the thought that I would not have to live alone anymore. We began to talk of renting a house in Northridge, near the state university. But it certainly wasn't a done deal. In fact, Mary almost bailed out on New Year's Eve after we'd agreed to spend the night at her place in Hollywood. I brought my recently completed whale costume with me. Our plan was to walk Hollywood Boulevard until midnight and check out the various parties.

The evening started out fine, but within blocks of her apartment I began to lose it. The problem was, with my ungainly costume on, I stood over seven feet tall and was nearly seven feet around the middle. To make matters worse, I could barely see through the slit in Willy's mouth; this made it impossible to anticipate where any curbs were located. Without asking Mary whether she wanted to, I appointed her to be my seeing-eye person, then began complaining bitterly every time I tripped over a curb.

The reason she decided not to send me and my whale costume packing back to Santa Monica was because people started to grow curious about the massive killer whale stumbling through the streets. We even got invited into a couple of parties. As the night progressed, Mary began laughing hilariously whenever I'd grow disoriented in the middle of a crosswalk and begin spinning around. Eventually, we trekked far enough that Mary desperately suggested we take a bus back to her place. The ride back gave her some time to relax and make sense of my all-too-boorish behavior. Her frustration proved to be a harbinger of stress to come, but Mary brushed it aside. She wanted this to work as much as I did.

Once we climbed off the bus, she invited me inside. Mary sat on the bed waiting for me to shed my Willy costume, a feat that almost threw me into another rage. I nearly destroyed the damn thing trying to pull it off. By the time I joined Mary on the bed, I was a sweaty mess. We made love, fell asleep, then I awoke next to her on New Year's morning. When I opened my eyes, the sun was in the process of creeping in through her bedroom window, bathing her back in a golden beam of light. Two of her birds were nestled between her shoulder blades. What a heavenly image, I thought, reaching my hand out and gently touching her skin with my open palm. I snuggled up to her and ran a few numbers and dates through my head. The two of us had met in 1993 and Mary would soon turn thirty-nine. Her next birthday would fall on a Sunday, just like her birthdate—and just like my last birthday had fallen on a Thursday, which was the day I was born.

New Year's Day went from good to great, morphing into one of the best days of my life. For starters, I didn't have that confounded Willy costume to stress me out. We watched football most of the day. Nobody had ever explained football to Mary, but she picked it up in a flash and actually enjoyed it. We shared peanut butter sandwiches with Ricky and Lucy, her two cockatiels, then set off for a nine-mile walk and grabbed a hamburger. I could have walked to Japan with Mary.

Oddly, I didn't want to go home. Usually, the end of any date I'd ever been on was tinged with awkwardness. I was either given the standard "I have to go home now." Or if I'd scored, I was the one who slipped away into the night, feeling like some sexual thief. But that wasn't the case on January 1, 1994. For the first time in my life, I felt wanted. And I knew that I wanted to keep this person in my life forever, as I still do.

In the days that followed, our relationship continued to grow deeper, far deeper than anything I'd ever imagined before. I was constantly burning to know everything going on inside her head and dying to share with her what was happening inside mine. Yet despite all the bliss, I was plagued by a single gnawing insecurity I just couldn't shake. Surely, any day now, Mary would wake up and realize what a mistake she'd made. Then what? Our mutual dream would wither. Every time we arranged to meet, the butterflies in my stomach nearly made me vomit. I'd hustle down to the bus stop a few blocks from my apartment, nervous as hell until I spotted her get off. And if for some reason she was late, I'd be thrown into even more of a panic. She's not coming, I'd tell myself. It's all over.

But Mary always showed up, although I didn't always recognize her at first because she'd often be wearing a different style of wig.

On the second weekend in January, Mary arrived at my apartment on a Friday. We goofed around for the next two days, seeing movies, watching TV, walking along the beach. On Sunday, we attended the monthly AGUA meeting. Afterward, we decided to stretch the weekend out one more night and Mary came back home with me. I figured we'd catch her bus across the city on Monday morning and I'd jump off within walking distance of my courier driving job. She'd continue on to her apartment in Hollywood.

But I wasn't needed at work on the morning of Monday, January 17, 1994, for the simple reason that a massive earthquake had turned Los Angeles upside down. Just 93 days after I'd met Mary in 1993, the two of us were shaken out of our sleep by a long, gut-rattling tremor. We threw our arms around each other as we bounced up and down upon the bed and watched our dove, New Dovenant, flutter out of her cast-iron cage to a curtain rod, seconds before the cage bounced across my dresser and tumbled onto the floor. After what seemed like hours, the shaking stopped and we waited for my screeching cockatiels to stop their panicked flapping and return to the unstable earth.

"What if that was centered in the ocean?" queried Mary. "We better get away from here."

Since we were only a few blocks from the Pacific, I had to admit that she was right. Ten minutes later, we were wandering down the street to a nearby bus stop, toting several birdcages and whatever clothes we could grab shoved in grocery bags. It wasn't the kind of night where bus drivers cared if passengers had wings, scales, or tails. The only thing on anyone's mind was getting to higher land.

The Northridge earthquake so trashed Mary's apartment that we decided she might as well move in with me. I could tell her two sons, both in their twenties, weren't too crazy about the idea of their mother embarking on what they believed would soon descend into yet another ill-fated romantic adventure. But they also saw how excited the two of us were, so they rolled with it. Mary lovingly referred to my place as a biohazard—not to be cute, but because it was the term that most accurately described it.

The morning after she moved in, I left for my courier job and she sprang into action. Stacks of newspapers, magazines, and notebooks filled with my writings sprouted from the floor of my apartment like mushrooms. Much of the place was coated with a layer of thick black dust or acrid piles of bird poop. I'd been unable to summon the nerve to throw anything away in years, and the place resembled a city dump. Yet despite the horrible mess, I knew where everything was. It was my world—chaotic, random, disheveled—but there was also a strange order to it. I didn't blame Mary for wanting to clean the place up—after all, there was a decomposing cockatiel in my closet.

Mary looked exhausted when I arrived home from work that night. The moment I opened the door and glanced around the front room, I sensed trouble brewing.

"What happened in here?" I stammered, gazing out at several recently decimated piles of newspaper. "Where's all my stuff?"

I felt dizzy, totally disoriented; the muscles in my neck were tensing. If I'd had a cork implanted in the top of my head, it would have popped out and embedded itself in the ceiling.

"Jerry," she laughed, grabbing hold of my hand. "I want you to meet your bathroom."

I was anything but amused, but I allowed myself to be pulled down the hall anyway, all the way to the bathroom, where she proudly showed me how she'd liberated the room from its coating of grime.

"This is your bathtub," she told me, pointing into the sparkling white porcelain tub. I stared at it in perplexed silence.

"And this is your toilet," she laughed. "Notice how it's no longer encrusted in brown fecal matter."

"Why did you do this?" I shouted. "Who told you to make all these changes?"

A fury swept through me like a hurricane. I felt possessed, angry, like I might pass out. As I began shrieking at her, she stomped out of the apartment. Still enraged but feeling like an absolute jerk, I ran to the window and watched as she marched down the sidewalk. I knew where she was going—to the nearby bluffs overlooking the ocean, where we'd shared our first kiss. By the time she returned, I'd cooled down.

"You didn't tell me you were going to do this," I muttered, digging through a stack of newspapers, searching for some obscure article I feared had probably been pitched into the garbage. "You have to tell me first when you do things like this ... when you do anything." I rubbed my hands frantically through my hair, staring down at the dirty carpet.

"I don't like surprises," I added, although I suppose I really didn't have to.

"Okay," she replied. "I promise. No more surprises ... But, Jerry, tomorrow when you get back from work, I swear to God that at least half of this apartment is going to be out in the Dumpster. That is, of course, unless you have a problem with that." She flashed me her most devilish, feminine grin.

What could I say to that? Mary was tweaking my universe and I was powerless to stop her. As much as I'd heard that love could conquer all, I never imagined it powerful enough to make me want to overcome my distaste for change.

Having never lived with a woman other than my mother, this new life of mine definitely took some getting used to. But one thing that didn't take long to get accustomed to was coming back to my apartment each night to this woman with an endless supply of wigs, who always had dinner simmering on the stove. We'd tell each other ridiculous stories, happy to have finally found each other after what seemed like several lifetimes spent searching. Her two boys were still on the fence about my role in Mary's life. They'd seen their mother hurt by too many men. Yet as our relationship deepened, our cockatiels also began growing closer and becoming a unified flock. Quite literally.

One afternoon, I walked into the bedroom and glimpsed Mary's bird, Ricky, and Pagliacci, whom I'd owned for years, standing together on my dresser, staring into the mirror. Without a moment's hesitation, I dumped a cup of bird seed on top of the dresser. Mary walked in just in time to watch them start devouring the seed.

"Look," I said. "They're doing lunch."

We both stood there laughing, feeling like the two luckiest people in the universe—alone but no longer lonely. Despite all the odds, all our idiosyncratic quirks, all the alienation we'd endured, we'd each finally found a friend, someone who understood, someone who could spend a half hour watching two birds munching sunflower seeds off the top of a cluttered dresser.

It was almost too much. And yet, in the midst of all this newfound bliss, there was also a heavy awkwardness. In many ways, we were like any other new couple learning the steps of that frustrating dance called living with your lover. Yet, what truly made the situation even more tense was my explosive temper. Try as I might, I often just couldn't control it. And the longer we lived together, the more I transformed myself into a walking land mine. All Mary had to do was brush up against me the wrong way and, with ever-increasing frequency, I'd detonate.

What was behind those ear-splitting outbursts? Part of the problem stemmed from my unwavering insistence that every single detail in my life be planned out. I hated surprises, loathed the unknown. Mary was the opposite. All her life, she had relied on fate and chance to guide her; she thrived on suspense.

Another source of my anger stemmed from my job. I felt trapped in it. Years before, I'd managed to convince myself that working as a courier driver represented a major step up from driving cabs. But after a couple of years, I was burned out, bitter, and depressed. I didn't want Mary to have to spend the rest of her life depending on a delivery driver to provide for her. Even more frustrating, because of AGUA I felt like I was closer than ever to actually achieving something with my life. And yet I was hopelessly mired in another dead-end job that was taking me nowhere.

My frustration came to a head one evening when Mary and I were riding a city bus across town and I suddenly realized that on the bus we'd just transferred from I'd left a folder filled with notes I'd made during a recent autism meeting. I panicked and jumped off the bus we were on, located a pay phone, and frantically dialed the number for the bus company, demanding that they find a dispatcher to contact the driver of that bus in order to locate my notes. After a half hour spent shrieking into the receiver, I gave up. Mary watched me from afar. She knew better than to get too close when I was having one of my grand mal tantrums. I slammed down the phone, walked over to a nearby curb, plopped myself down onto the concrete, and began to sob quietly. Mary inched closer, then she sat beside me on the curb.

"Is this all there is to my life?" I moaned. "I want us to have so much more than this, but nothing I do seems to change anything. I can't even help myself, let alone other people."

I felt Mary wrap her arm around me and lean the side of her head against mine. She wasn't wearing a wig, so I could feel the prickles of her closely shorn scalp. She didn't say anything. Not a single word. Yet she had a way of listening that spoke volumes. I always wished I had the ability to listen like that when Mary came to me with her problems, to be supportive in that sort of unspoken way. But I couldn't. All I could offer were my ears and she needed more than that. She needed exactly what she was giving me on that horrible evening when I felt the world closing in around me. With Mary's powerful arm draped around me, it didn't take long before I noticed that my breathing had slowed and the blinding rage inside my head had faded. I no longer felt so splintered and angry. A strange sense of peace came over me. Maybe that's why Mary kept her head on my shoulder, why the two of us just sat there with the city's evening rush-hour traffic roaring past us, inches from our toes, breathing the sweetest-smelling exhaust either of us had ever taken into our lungs.

By the spring of 1994, Mary had landed a job in a medical library at UCLA. Not long after starting, thanks to her incessant lobbying (which she never told me about until years later) of her boss at UCLA, Dr. Linda Deemer, I managed to get an interview at the financial office in the university's medical center. Dr. Deemer, who was raised in Tucson near where Mary grew up, had an autistic son. She helped me arrange an interview with my future boss, Gail Chorna, which resulted in my getting yet another glimpse at how my Asperger's mind processed information. A few minutes into the interview with Gail, she told me how surprised she was that I didn't recognize her.

"Don't you remember?" she laughed. "We met at my aunt's Christmas party. I came with my nephew, Byron. He's autistic."

"You weren't dressed like you are now," I apologized. "You were wearing holiday attire. . . . That's what threw me. That's what always throws me when I meet someone in a different setting and their plumage is different than it was when I last met them."

Gail seemed truly intrigued by the way my brain worked, and she eventually hired me as an administrative assistant in the med school's financial office. She wanted to give me the chance that she—and her family—hoped someone would someday give her nephew. She wanted him to have a life. I thanked Gail for the job, but I've always wished I'd told her that, with a family like hers, she didn't need to worry about her Byron. He'd always have a life.

Learning that I'd actually landed the job made me feel like a new man. I telephoned Mary and told her the good news. She pretended to be surprised, making me believe I'd gotten the position totally on my own. My coworkers were happy for me, too. They no longer had to wonder why I was driving a delivery car, instead of working at a place like UCLA. But the biggest boost that my new job gave me was permission to dream, to visualize a future for myself that had always seemed out of reach when I was trapped in a job I'd long ago begun to loathe. It proved to be the final piece in the puzzle that I needed to make the great leap—to convince myself that becoming someone's husband might not be that far-fetched an idea.

On the last day of April, I showed up at our apartment and told Mary there was something I needed to say to her. She smiled and tried to pretend she had no idea what I was talking about. We hopped a bus and rode to a nearby church with a massive fig tree growing out front. Whenever I'd driven past it during the course of my courier job, it never ceased to put me in a good mood. Its enormous size boggled my mind. Its reported age was numerically pleasing. It certainly seemed like a magical spot to ask someone to marry me, so that's what I decided to do.

"I think the two of us have something very unusual," I told Mary, holding her hand in mine. "And I'd like to make it last as long as possible."

Mary shouted, "I will!"

Three months later, in August, we got married in a church just up the street from where Nicole Brown Simpson had been stabbed to death earlier in the summer. Standing there beside Mary in that nearly empty church, I desperately wanted to pinch myself. Looking back on the moment, I wish I had. Maybe it would have woken me up.

HOLLYWOOD, CALIFORNIA
DECEMBER 1993

Six weeks after that day when Jerry dressed up as the world's largest mammal and I pretended to be one of history's most famous musicians, it happened. We embarked upon our first date. Jerry wanted to take me to the horse races, but I quickly nixed the idea because neither of us owned a car and getting there seemed like a logistical nightmare. So we went to the Los Angeles County

Zoo instead. Jerry showed up at my apartment in an ill-fitting T-shirt with smears of ketchup on it. I tried not to dwell on it, but over the next hour, as we rode one city bus after another, I found myself transfixed by the bloodred stains. I thought it resembled a piece of modern art.

During our bus ride, we talked about everything—or at least attempted to. At one point, I tried to recount the latest soap opera unfolding within my family and how it was affecting me. But Jerry just looked at me as though he had no earthly idea why I was sharing this information with him. I felt myself grow angry, but calmed myself down because there was something so honest about him. Jerry didn't candy-coat a thing. He just flat out told me I sounded like a lunatic. (The only other person I'd ever heard make such a ridiculously honest statement was when I sometimes opened my mouth.) The farther we traveled in that bus, the more Jerry opened up to me. As the buildings and billboards rolled past the dirty windows, he revealed his bitterness over never being able to put his mathematical talents to use.

"I feel like I've wasted a gift I never even wanted," he moaned. "And now it's too late."

"I know exactly what you mean," I told him, feeling as though we were two parts of the same sponge. All I wanted to do was soak him up.

The shadows were sharp and short on that sunny November afternoon. That was always how I remembered the time of year when something occurred in my life—by thinking back to the length of the shadows during a certain time of a specific day. The place was practically empty as we wandered from one exhibit to the next, spending most of our time staring at the birds and monkeys. Jerry's ability to look at an animal and transform it into a cartoon caricature fascinated me. He seemed to ooze whimsy, which was contrasted with the heavy, objective way I often viewed the world, one of my inheritances from my scientific-minded parents.

Two hours after arriving, we hopped another bus and began the long ride back to my apartment. Unfortunately, I put us on the wrong bus, which meant we ended up hoofing it a couple of miles to catch the appropriate ride. This induced a minor temper tantrum in Jerry, who walked behind me, grumbling and moaning over my ineptitude. I tried to ignore him. I tried to write off his foul temper to autism, doing my best to convince myself that his rage was caused by something apart from him, something entirely separate. I desperately didn't want this beautiful day to end on such an ugly, discordant note.

Time stumbled onward and with it came the realization that Jerry didn't have a scrap of the experience that I had in relationships. He told me that he hadn't had a girlfriend—or anything closely resembling one—in more than a decade and hadn't ventured out on a date for almost five years. But his naïveté didn't bother me. I thought it was sweet—at least at first I did. It was clear from the start that Jerry did a lot of thinking on the topic of us having sex. Yet for all that mental energy he put into it, he was so very insecure in bed. Part of it had to do with his anatomy.

When God handed out penises, Jerry must have been standing at the end of the line, counting railcars or crunching numbers. He took a lot of grief due to his plumbing when he was young and I knew this topic still bothered him—a lot more than I imagined it would ever bother me. But what did I know? I grew up as a girl with Asperger's. We have it far easier than guys do. All we have to do is fix up our hair and put on some nice clothes and voilà! We're suddenly sexy. We just aren't held to the same standards that guys are. We're just kooky girls with great hair, wardrobes, and bodies.

Jerry was also amazingly ignorant about anything having to do with intimacy. His idea of sex was to have it, then get it over as soon as possible. He had no clue about what was going on down there from my side of the action. For someone as smart as he was, I couldn't understand why he never consulted a book on comparative anatomy. I was naïve enough to believe that this wouldn't always be the case. And I was certainly willing to give him time as long as other parts of our relationship made up for this deficiency.

Which was certainly the case—at first.

Back then, every day with Jerry felt like I was walking though an amusement park. We shared literally every silly thing that percolated through our heads. Our place was a constant mess. But with all of our birds flapping about, it was also quite blissful. We possessed a sense of humor that tended to see levity where most people cannot. We could stare at our birds for hours, giggling whenever they made a funny expression or fluffed up their feathers in a silly way. We didn't have to do expensive things and go on big dates to keep the interest alive between us. Just being together with someone who viewed the world the way I did was more than enough.

After I moved into Jerry's apartment, the days started to blend together like some strange casserole. We fell into a routine like any other couple would. Each morning, Jerry went off to work and I'd stay home, cleaning, sometimes reading the poetry, musings, and doodlings that he'd filled his notebooks with. It was an idyllic few months. Sometimes, I'd draw or paint. Before long, however, the bliss gave way to my worst fears. Once the novelty of bedding me had died away, Jerry reverted back to the hypersensitive person he must have been before we met. He morphed into a sensory porcupine, which made living with him pure hell. I tiptoed around him most of the time. The minute he got on the phone or started wading through his e-mail, he became a man possessed, completely intolerant of any distraction. The fun aspect of our relationship, the sharing of our two walled worlds, began to slip away and was soon replaced by a lukewarm cold war.

The fact that it never occurred to me to cut and run wasn't surprising. After all, I'd stuck it out in far worse relationships. But all those other men were acting like macho pigs because ... well, they *were* macho pigs. Jerry, however, was different. His boorish behavior really did emanate from his autism—just like much of the workings of his mind did. I could either choose to accept that, as he had accepted my shortcomings. Or I could pack up my belongings and hit the road.

One afternoon in April, Jerry and I hopped a city bus and headed up National Boulevard to a church I'd never seen before. I pretended I didn't know what he was up to, but it was obvious. He took me to an ancient fig tree that—because of its age—held some special numerical meaning for him. It felt ancient, the way its graceful ancient trunk twisted and turned upward into the sky. But instead of being impressed by it, I felt uneasy when I saw how shriveled and unappetizing its purplish figs were. It reminded me of a similar tree that Jesus once cursed because it didn't bring forth good fruit. Nevertheless, I loved the way Jerry was able to weave together how all the numbers relating to this tree paralleled our two lives. Everywhere he looked, he saw numbers. And on that day it felt like he was painting a portrait out of them.

The week after our engagement proved to be a magical time for our birds, too. My two cockatiels—Ricky and Lucy—hatched their first chick, Wolfgang, beneath our cluttered bed. I'll never forget the sensation of gently placing the little pink fellow into my hand and marveling at the sensation his strong legs made as they pushed down into my palm. So spindly, but filled with such life. Wolfgang grew up quickly and was flying within five weeks, singing nonstop. Jerry and I used to love watching Wolfgang socializing with the others on the dresser, curtain rod, and bedroom door. His occasional expeditions into the kitchen and living room were often the highlight of our week. Who needed TV when you have a home filled with cockatiels? Because of his father's industrial-strength libido, we had to separate Wolfgang from Ricky for several months, which broke our hearts. Ricky would literally mount any cockatiel in sight, male or female, and used his feeding duties as an excuse to try to mount his newborn son.

When I first brought Lucy home to our apartment, Ricky immediately mounted her without even an introduction. I'd known a few men like that, so I explained to Lucy how she didn't have to put up with it. She must have listened to my advice because she always rejected Ricky's uncouth advances and it took her a long time to forgive him. But Ricky was incredibly friendly, with the type of squinty eyes that reminded everyone of a pirate. His favorite activity, besides humping things, was to climb on Jerry's shoulder and groom him, picking at the stubble on his cheek.

It didn't take a psychiatrist to realize that Jerry and I doted on our birds as though they were our children. Ricky was eight. Lucy, a sweet yellow and white lutino, was six. Jerry's oldest cock, Pagliacci, who was ten years old, had a crush on Lucy from the moment he first laid eyes on her. But because Pagliacci and Ricky were friends, Lucy was safe from his advances. Then there was Isadora Duncan, almost five. She was the first chick hatched in Jerry's home, a truly blessed event that occurred several years before we met. And finally, there was four-year-old Cockatiel Dundee. He was the spitting double of his dad, although with a slightly larger crest that he seemed particularly proud of, judging by the way he'd parade around the apartment showing it to everyone.

One day, a woman showed up at the pet shop where my son Peter worked in Santa Monica, carrying a young white-faced female named Sylvia. We adopted her and suddenly Cockatiel Dundee had a nonrelated single female to fixate on. Sylvia, however, was so behind in her bird socialization skills that I called her my "shoulder potato," since all she wanted to do was perch on my shoulder all day.

"Maybe she's autistic," Jerry suggested.

"She'll catch on," I replied, feeling protective of my newest daughter.

After a few months of seeing how happy all our cockatiels were, we began to feel sorry for our sole dove, New Dovenant. She looked so lonely that Jerry eventually tracked down a "mail-order husband," for her, whom we named Eternal Dovenant. Our new male, however, seemed slow to grasp the physical requirement of his job as a hired stud. New Dovenant, however, wasn't about to let this little technicality stop her. She stalked her new man around the house, showing him her butt at every opportunity. A few days later, he finally understood what was expected of him. He began shimmying up and down like Chubby Checker on *American Bandstand* and soon went to work on his mate.

And so, shortly after Jerry and I were engaged, our bird families were all celebrating new additions to their little groups. Winged or not, the future looked bright for all of us.

Not long after we moved in together, I managed to land a job in the biomedical library at UCLA, working for Dr. Linda Deemer, a cardiology professor from my hometown of Tucson, who had an autistic son. All day long, I'd pull research papers for her on everything from thrombosis and scar tissue to cellular intelligence and arrhythmia, periodically reading the articles in order to absorb all the information I could before delivering the material to various doctors. I never knew it was possible to feel so mentally stimulated in a job. Yet I also couldn't help imagining how I would have felt if I hadn't been so drugged up. I'd recently been diagnosed with epilepsy, so I'd begun taking a number of powerful medications to ward off any potential seizures. On top of that, ever since cleaning out Jerry's apartment I'd begun experiencing debilitating migraines. The only remedy involved popping a combination of potent painkillers whenever I felt one coming on.

As our wedding day inched closer, I'd become a listless, walking zombie. I asked myself over and over, Why am I marrying this man? How did all this happen so quickly? Would I really be going through all this if my life hadn't been so insane? I thought back to when Jerry and I first met, back to when I was still licking my wounds from my last failed romance, contemplating homicide. Jerry's wonderfully clueless interest in me and his approach to dating not only were refreshing, but also distracted me from all that pain and hurt. Yet the sexiest thing of all was the way he put me up on a pedestal and treated me like I was something special. No man had ever done that.

So why did I say yes when Jerry proposed? Was I sure it would work? Not at all. But I felt honored that Jerry had never even taken this chance before, yet he was willing to take it with me. I said yes, hoping it would work but also feeling that Jerry deserved a chance at marriage. In his clueless but sincere way, he yearned to be a hero for me. So I figured I'd give him a shot at doing just that.

Besides, what could I lose other than time?

And on the afternoon the two of us stood beside each other in that church in Westwood, the sun burned bright, the shadows were medium length, and I wore a black velvet vest made in Thailand and covered with elephants. As the minister said a few words about the transformative powers of love, I stood there gripping Jerry's arm tightly, wondering if this was all just a crazy dream. Somewhere inside my head, I imagined myself deep underwater, far below the surface of the sea. Peter and Steve sat behind us in a pew, no doubt wondering what their nutty mother was up to now. I tried to smile, but the medication had deadened my facial nerves.

When it was all over and Jerry and I had become man and wife, we climbed onto a city bus and rode to the Santa Monica pier, where we ate our grocery-store-bought wedding cake. The sticker on the box promised it was a carrot cake, which had been my favorite ever since childhood. Jerry, however, kept referring to it as a "parrot cake." I was in no shape to know the difference. And since the strange combination of drugs I'd been ingesting over the past few months had killed off my taste buds, all I could do was chew the soft lump in my mouth and try to remember.

Chapter Eight

Although our relationship began to self-destruct a month after our wedding, the real problems started on that morning Mary bulldozed her way through my apartment, trying to clean up the mess it had taken me years to make. Not long afterward, she began complaining about terrible headaches and a lack of energy. She eventually developed pneumonia-like symptoms and had to be taken to the hospital. Her lungs were barely working. For more than a week she just lay there in bed, staring at the avocado-tinted wall. That electric spark I'd fallen in love with had vanished right in front of my eyes. The doctors finally allowed her to return to our apartment, but she was there for only a few hours before her symptoms returned and she needed to be rushed back to the hospital. I felt horrible, thinking that my mess was responsible for her ill health, and eventually we found another apartment located a couple of miles away.

But by then, we were already on a collision course for trouble. Mary's health improved a bit, but she continued to remain listless. Before long, she'd quit her job, claiming that the bright lights from the photocopy machine were inducing epileptic seizures. Day by day, it was as if a brick wall were being erected between us. (Then again, perhaps it was only being rebuilt after we'd both allowed it to be torn down during those first blissful months of our relationship.) Before long, we'd stopped talking about anything of real importance. Looking back on it, should I really have expected things to have been any different? After all, I had no experience or appreciation of intimacy. Instead of sharing, I kept everything locked and hidden inside my head and heart. And it stayed there, just below the surface, simmering. Every so often, when something trivial happened, such as when Mary turned the TV volume up too loud or when she decided to move a stack of my newspapers, all that emotion I'd kept clamped up inside me would explode out of me, usually in a fit of angry rage.

Back then, my performance seemed perfectly natural. After all, I told myself that since I'd married someone just like me, I could behave any way I wanted. Which was why, only a year into our relationship, I reverted back to my old, touchy self. I was *just* being me, *just* being Jerry. So when Mary would accidentally brush up against me, it seemed perfectly normal to scream at her. And if I bumped my toe against a chair, I didn't think twice about shrieking at the top of my lungs.

Mary, of course, had her own term for my outbursts. "You're barking again," she'd tell me.

To which I'd roar: "Well, at least I don't hit you."

Whenever I'd make a comment like that, the look Mary got on her face always seemed to express the same thought: being hit couldn't be any worse than how I was treating her.

Needless to say, our lovemaking sessions soon turned into an empty ritual that Mary tolerated but obviously didn't enjoy. Who could blame her? Once, when we were lying in bed, she thought it would be funny to press her lips up against my chest and start blowing, making faux fart noises. As was typical, I exploded.

"Don't do that!" I screamed. "Don't touch me like that!"

Mary didn't shout back. She rarely did that back then. She'd just shut down, much like that robot on *Lost in Space* when someone yanked the power pack out of his neck. She'd roll over and curl into a fetal ball.

"I need to be alone, Jerry," she'd whisper.

Which, of course, was the last thing I ever allowed her to do. Instead of giving her some space to breathe, I'd blast into hyperdrive, clumsily trying to fix the situation right then and there by ranting and raving, trying to force her to understand my side of things. And this only made the situation worse.

I just didn't get it. I was suffering from terminal cluelessness.

By the summer of 1995, Mary was clearly ready to leave our marriage. I could see her desire to be finished with our relationship whenever I dared look into her eyes. Then it happened. One day in July when I was away at work, the telephone rang at our apartment. A *Los Angeles Times* reporter named Kim Kowsky told us she wanted to write a story on autism. She'd heard about Mary and me and wanted to interview us for an article she was writing. Why not? we thought. If nothing else, it would be nice to get a bit of publicity for our group. So we met Kim a handful of times. She even attended an AGUA gathering.

A few months later, on October 23, the 296th day of the year, her story finally made it into print. Only instead of being buried in the back of the newspaper, it appeared on the front page. The headline read: "Against the Odds: A Love Story." Instead of focusing on AGUA, the article centered on the two of us. Before we knew it, the phone in our apartment started ringing. People I hadn't spoken to in years were calling. It seemed the whole world had read that article. Within a couple of days, the power brokers in Hollywood smelled a feature film in our quirky love story. Suddenly, we were the most popular kids on the playground. It felt like every producer and director in town wanted to be our new friend. My phone at work and in our apartment began ringing incessantly. It didn't take long before I got caught up in the hoopla and the attention, convincing myself that I was someone bigger and more important than I really was, that the world needed to hear *my* story.

We ended up signing a deal with a top Hollywood agent, who had the corner office at the town's most powerful talent agency. Rumors were afloat that Robin Williams wanted to play me in the movie. Suddenly, all the insurmountable problems that Mary and I were experiencing with our relationship became just a bit more tolerable. A movie meant money—possibly big money. It didn't take long before I convinced myself that if we had a chunk of cash in the bank, it might actually take some of the angry, desperate edge off our relationship.

So we played the game.

Hollywood resembled an inexplicable parallel universe, the kind of strange dimension where Mary's Bolian character on *Star Trek* would have felt quite at home. One minute the negotiations behind our movie were moving forward at the speed of light. The next, they had creaked to a standstill. During one of those chaotic stints, our agent telephoned to say that Steven Spielberg wanted to "take a meeting" with us. A few weeks before, Spielberg had bought a spec script to our story for an unprecedented $2.5 million after outbidding several other studios.

"And Robin Williams will be there," our agent added. "He wants to meet the two of you."

So I took the day off from work. The assistant to Ron Bass, the *Rain Man* screenwriter hired to pen our movie script, drove us to Spielberg's DreamWorks office. We were both excited. Mary even brought Shayna, our prized Goffin's cockatoo, along for the meeting. Immediately after arriving, Spielberg's secretary shepherded us into an empty boardroom.

After a half hour spent waiting, I started to panic. So much was riding on this meeting, I told myself. Try as I might, I couldn't understand what was keeping them. Had they lost interest in us? It reminded me of all those times in college I anxiously waited for one of my dates to appear, nauseated by the possibility that I'd been stood up. I wanted to kick myself. How could I let myself get so caught up in all this Hollywood nonsense? I began to doubt if we'd even get a free lunch out of the deal. My mood grew dark. Eventually, Steven and Robin appeared. They couldn't have been nicer.

"Hey, Jerry . . . Mary," Steven said. "I want you two to meet Robin Williams. He's really interested in this project."

Quite naturally, the first thing I did was ask Robin when he was born. He told me and I immediately performed my number-crunching birthday trick. Shayna, who was the two-winged incarnation of Bart Simpson, lunged at Steven and managed to tear a button off his shirt. While Mary wrestled the button out of Shayna's beak, it dawned on me that Robin was born 1,066 days before me.

"The year 1066 was a big one for William the Conqueror," I announced. "Maybe you can conquer this role." The two men laughed, shook our hands, and disappeared down the hallway. Our big meeting was over. And, before I knew it, so was my love affair with Hollywood. As much as I hated to admit it, I'd begun to grow tired of the roller-coaster ride. Wondering exactly who was going to portray me in our much-heralded movie had lost its appeal. And from what I'd seen of Tinseltown, I had a hunch that even if the film did get made, we probably wouldn't even recognize our own story.

A few weeks later, our agent arranged for us to appear on *60 Minutes*. By then, however, all the giddiness and excitement surrounding our fifteen minutes' worth of fame had faded. Mary and I had fallen back into our tired old routine. I'd explode, Mary would withdraw, and then I'd hound her, trying to make everything better. Most days, after I'd go to work, Mary never bothered leaving the apartment. If she could muster up the energy, she'd paint. Much of the time, she just stayed in bed. Still, she had this sexuality that oozed from her. And her body had the uncanny ability to change shape depending on her mood—one minute she was taut and slender, the next chubby. She reminded me of our cockatiels. They could either puff their feathers up to make themselves seem larger or pull them tight against their body, creating a look of sheer sleekness.

Shortly before the TV camera crews descended on us, Mary convinced me that we should move to a bigger place. I agreed, partly out of guilt over the havoc my temper had been wreaking on our relationship, partly because I believed that getting a house would somehow keep things alive and help diffuse some of the tension between us, since we both would have our own bedroom. So, in June of 1996, we packed up our menagerie and moved into the largest house I'd ever lived in. It was also the most expensive. Instead of saving what little windfall we'd netted from Hollywood, we were spending it almost as quickly as the checks arrived in the mail.

As if Mary and I didn't have enough problems, it was around this time that my Internet addiction began destroying what little calm remained in our lives. Ever since I'd discovered cyberspace, I'd had a serious issue with not being able to control my temper when I was online. When I think back on the whole situation and the way I got so fixated and worked up over the stupidest stuff, it now seems so very autistic of me. Of course, I couldn't see that back then. It all started when Mary and I began logging on to a few Internet lists devoted to autism and "meeting" other people. For a while, the experience was fun for both of us.

The problem, of course, was me. Not long after I discovered the World Wide Web, I got into a feud with somebody from another list that began to consume me. I would wake up at any hour of night, log on, and send e-mails to support my side of the never-ending verbal battle we were waging. I should have let it go, but I couldn't—especially back then. The argument revolved around a claim that somebody from my support group had made, which apparently convinced some people on the East Coast that AGUA was a kind of MENSA for autistics, that only savants were allowed to join. Not only wasn't that true, it hurt me to think that anyone would believe I'd run such a ridiculous group, which would exclude so many of my current AGUA members. Why on earth had I continued to state my case when anyone who actually showed up for an AGUA meeting could see how absurd this person's claim was?

Once at a conference we both attended, Mary asked the woman who had sparked this mini-controversy why she'd told this lie. She quickly replied, "I need people to believe this, so I can a write a book."

Mary patted her on the back, then smiled at me and shook her head. "No one is ever going to publish her book, Jerry," she whispered a few minutes later. "You really need to forget about this."

Of course I need to, I thought to myself. But I can't.

Instead, I continued to fume and rant over my computer keyboard. It was just so important for me to be right, so absolutely critical that my voice be heard and accepted. And so I continued my late-night flame war with my cyber foe. The only problem was that every time I'd log on, I'd wake Mary up. She'd lie there in bed and listen to me pounding away on the keyboard, cursing to myself over the latest insult hurled my way, then she'd whisper, "Why are you doing this to yourself, Jerry? Why are you doing this to us?"

For the longest time, I could not come up with an answer to her question. But there was something about Mary's patience with me that caused me to believe that someday I would know the answer. Within a few months, I finally got a good look at myself, realizing how I was behaving like an idiot, how I'd blown this whole issue so out of proportion. I was not only embarrassed over the truly stupid stuff I'd been writing, I felt guilty that I'd allowed it to inject so much insanity into our home life.

It's been more than ten years now since all that silliness. In that time, I've met and made friends with many of my former targets and attackers during my days as an e-mail warrior. I've also adopted a few rules that I've tried to follow:

1. Resist the temptation to check my e-mail at home.
2. Wait twenty-four hours before responding to *any* offensive message.
3. Before sending any message that might offend a group, run it by somebody who understands the context in which that group might read it.

These rules aren't perfect, but they definitely make my e-mail time a lot more productive and fun—not to mention a lot less destructive. But even more important, every time I log on to a computer, I'm reminded of Mary and the patience she exhibited when cyber rage was tearing me apart. Deep down she understood what I was going through and believed in me enough to trust that I'd finally find my way back to sanity.

Few things in life happen without a reason. For those who keep their eyes open, there are precious few surprises. If you watch closely enough, everything happens as the result of something else. Like dominoes falling, one after another, the events in one's life are merely a reaction to what came before it. One of those dominoes was my offer to let Mary's two sons live with us in the downstairs bedrooms of our newly rented home. Peter and Steve, both in their early twenties, were great guys who loved their mother in a way that went far deeper than anything I'd ever witnessed between a mother and her sons. The three of them had been through hell together and somehow survived intact. But Peter and Steve were also two young bucks, full of wild energy. I could just barely handle living with Mary. Adding her two sons into the mix quickly added one more ingredient to our recipe for disaster.

Initially, I think Peter and Steve truly wanted to like me, although they didn't quite know what to make of me. I definitely wasn't like any of the other guys their mother had been involved with. And despite all my explosive tendencies, I was definitely more stable than any of my predecessors. Even more important for her two boys, I sometimes seemed to be able to make their mother happy.

But as time went on, their opinion of me changed. Eventually, whatever respect they had for me was lost. I suppose I can't really blame them. The tipping point came one afternoon when the four of us were driving up to Santa Barbara to visit Mary's parents. Peter and Steve were sitting in the backseat. We were taking a shortcut and I unwittingly made Mary my copilot, entrusting her with our map and directions, scrawled on a piece of paper. All her life, Mary has always somehow managed to end up exactly where she needed to go, but the route she inevitably took was enough to induce an aneurysm in an obsessive veteran cabdriver such as myself. I now realize that, without meaning to, I'd set Mary up to fail. And when that happened, it was only a matter of time before my temper exploded with the ferocity of a car bomb, affecting anyone who happened to be within earshot of my voice.

On that particular afternoon, we were heading north out of Los Angeles. It didn't take long before things turned ugly.

"Don't I turn here?" I asked Mary, after spotting a street that I vaguely recognized as part of our route.

"Sure," Mary replied. "Why don't you turn here."

"But is that what's written on the directions?" I shouted, feeling my blood starting to boil.

"Sure, Jerry," she said. "It's on the directions, right here . . . somewhere." Mary paused for a moment, beginning to sound flustered as she read over the piece of paper I'd given her. "Well, I thought those were the directions. Go ahead and turn here and let's see what happens."

"But you can't do that, Mary!" I screamed, pulling over to the side of the road. "That's not how it works!"

"Jerry," she said with a nervous laugh. "We'll get there eventually. We always do."

And that was all it took. *Kabooooooooom!* I detonated. Mary flinched a bit at first, when the words hit her. But then a sort of glazed look fell over her and she just sat there and took all my acoustic punches, every last one. When it was all over and the rage had passed, I felt ashamed. Suddenly, I remembered her two sons sitting in the backseat. I sheepishly looked up into the rearview mirror and saw them both sitting there, grim-faced, staring straight ahead, boring holes into the back of my head. Years would pass before I finally realized that I wasn't yelling at Mary. I was yelling because that was what Jerry Newport did when his buttons got pushed. I was yelling because I'd long ago grown used to the sound of my own thunder. I was yelling because I didn't know how not to yell.

At least not yet I didn't.

Whenever she could muster up the energy, Mary did her artwork or composed music. I loved that she had something she was passionate about, something that made her feel alive. What frustrated me was that she continually brushed aside my suggestions that she should try to make some money from her creative gifts. I didn't know much about how she might have gone about marketing her creations, but her paintings were absolutely stunning. There was no reason, I thought, she couldn't sell them or find someone who'd do it for her.

"It's not the right time," she'd always tell me.

"What's that supposed to mean?" I'd shout. "It seems like all you're doing is *wasting* your time."

That would usually be the end of it. Mary would disappear into her bedroom, mumbling about how tired her medications made her, then she'd shut the door, desperately trying to avoid any discussion on the matter. And I'd just stand there thinking about how rough a city like Los Angeles can be on the delicate senses of someone like Mary . . . and on someone like me. Even more frustrating was that I felt partially responsible for her malaise. After all, I was the one who first suggested she begin seeing the physician who seemed content to pump her full of more and more drugs, none of which seemed to do any good.

Our role as media poster specimens also put an added strain on our relationship. We'd both spent a lifetime craving recognition, but now it seemed as though our notoriety was bringing out the worst in our Asperger's. This insatiable need to be heard over and above anyone else is definitely an Aspie trait. Why we were so blind to this fact, I just don't know. For example, one afternoon a reporter from *People* magazine dropped by to interview us. She flipped on her tape recorder and began asking Mary some questions. By the time she got done with her interrogation, she'd nearly run out of tape, which caused me to fly into a rage. This scenario repeated itself whenever a reporter, producer, or screenwriter happened to telephone us and whoever answered stayed on the line too long. Of course, my way of handling the situation was much more obnoxious than Mary's. I'd stomp around in front of her while she was talking on the phone and mimic the "cut" signal by dragging my index finger across my throat.

By the time the *60 Minutes* camera crews began tromping through our house, even I realized our relationship was in serious trouble. It seemed like only a matter of time before we went our separate ways.

Yet we didn't.

The *60 Minutes* piece aired in September and the hoopla started all over again. We'd become autism's "First Couple." The segment centered upon our much-hyped poignant and touching love for each other. At that time, it felt like most of this love existed only in the past tense. When it was all over and our segment finally aired, Mary and I sat there watching our images flicker across the TV screen. We didn't say a word to each other, but deep down we both knew we were feeling the same thing—dishonest. Like we'd both just told the biggest lie of our lives to millions of people. It wasn't a good feeling. Neither one of us was a good liar. Far from it. If anything, it was our maddening tendency toward brutal honesty that had wreaked so much havoc in our lives. Lies just weren't part of the program that we had running through our heads. To lie isn't autistic; it's a break from the order that our brains so badly crave.

Yet the two of us hung on to whatever it was that remained of our relationship. Did we stick it out because of fear? Or was it due to laziness? Perhaps it was a bit of both, with a touch of desperation thrown in. After all, I was in my midforties at the time. I told myself that I had to be out of my mind to believe I was ever going to find a woman without at least a few dings and dents.

Mostly, though, I accepted the way we were living because it confirmed everything I knew about relationships and love. After all, I'd grown up in a house where my parents slept in separate beds. Marriage wasn't an intimate thing. It was a long-term friendship, a cooperative coexistence. And no matter how far Mary tried to push me away, I continued to believe we could work it out.

Maybe I felt that way because I sometimes believed that the whole world was rooting for us to stay together. As crazy as it sounds, even in our darkest moments, we both could sense that our relationship was giving people hope, was helping them to believe that the human heart didn't have to be hampered by the wiring of the brain. But the truth was that no matter how angry I got with Mary, I couldn't shake her from my system. She'd managed to wedge herself inside me like a splinter that filled me with unimaginable ecstasy, but mostly—at least lately—just made me crazy. I'd never felt so connected to another person, so safe and cared for. At times, it seemed almost enough to override all the frustration we were experiencing.

Mary's health continued to spiral downward. She rarely left her bed and constantly complained of terrible blinding migraines. The doctors couldn't understand what could be behind her ailments. Eventually the specialists decided that a hysterectomy might be her best bet. One night, not long after her surgery and her return from the hospital, she wrote a one-page letter, laid it on her bed-side table, and when she was sure everyone had gone to sleep, she swallowed every pill she could get her hands on, literally hundreds of them, then crawled back into her bed.

I found her the next morning, barely breathing. Peter called the ambulance and she was rushed to a nearby hospital.

"Why didn't you let me go?" she demanded. "Why?"

When they finally allowed Mary to leave the hospital and return home, the atmosphere between us continued to deteriorate. We barely spoke, at least not about anything important. But even during the worst of times, we both held on to the idea that if our little story could help one person, could instill a bit of hope in the life of someone like us, someone lost who needed to find the way, then maybe everything we were going through would be worth it.

But by Valentine's Day of 1997, even that shared belief seemed like a ridiculous fantasy. Mary was out of bed that evening when I came home from work clutching a dozen roses, still bullheadedly hoping that we could make everything work out. When Mary saw the roses, she grabbed them out of my hands, buried her face in the bloodred petals, then hurled them across the room.

"I want a divorce." She laughed. "I want a divorce and I want you to get out."

All I could do was stare down at the floor, down at the random pattern the rose stems made on top of the carpet. The Ozzie and Harriet of autism, it seemed, would soon be going their separate ways.

Santa Monica, California
November 1994

I stopped singing to the birds.

That should have been my first clue that something was wrong. All my life, I'd hummed, whistled, and sung to whatever carbon-based entities were within earshot. Then one day, my little self-produced symphonies ceased. The only music I created was on paper. The air in our apartment was filled with nothing but silence and tension. The walls went up between us, those same walls that we'd so giddily torn down months before, back when we'd first met. Then again, maybe we'd never actually ripped anything down. Maybe we'd imagined the whole thing. Love will do that to you.

Whatever the reason, a few weeks into our marriage something became apparent: the monster that had chased me all my life had somehow tracked down my home address and was now camped out in our living room. Any delusions that love was going to transform my life into some happily-ever-after fairy tale had begun feeling like just another one of my ridiculous pipe dreams.

For someone who couldn't summon up the courage to part with a single piece of paper, Jerry didn't seem the least bit upset with having to leave the apartment where he and his mother had lived together for years. He did it for me, which I thought was sweet. No man had ever done something like that for me before. What did annoy him, however, was my deteriorating health. He hated it that the iron-bodied, rock-hard woman he'd fallen in love with, the one who used to enjoy going on hundred-mile bike rides through the San Gabriel Mountains, had become a physical wreck. But that's exactly what I'd become. If it wasn't the migraines, the vertigo, or the projectile vomiting, it was the painful pus-filled cysts that had begun to pop up beneath my skin like mushrooms. I tried to fight it, tried to will myself to make it all go away, but I couldn't—at least not for very long. Every so often I'd muster up enough strength to get back up on my feet and pretend that everything was okay, then I'd collapse back into bed for an entire week. That's when Jerry really began yelling at me. He was frustrated. I could see that. But I was helpless to do anything about it. And I hated feeling so powerless.

More than anything else, I couldn't stand Jerry's vocal attacks. I don't mind people yelling at me. I'd long ago perfected the art of tuning out hurtful words and transforming the cacophony into harmless white noise. Sometimes, however, instead of tuning the other person out, I actually listened to their rant and pondered their accusations. I'd mine their hurtful words and pluck out a nugget or two that I could apply toward my life, that I could use to transform myself into a better person. Yet what I couldn't handle were verbal beatings that had nothing to do with me or my short-comings, that were nothing more than groundless tirades. Besides, I possessed enough self-loathing to cripple ten people. Whatever denigrations Jerry hurled my way were bush league compared to the hate and hurt I inflicted upon myself every minute.

Nevertheless, when it came to explosions of anger, Jerry was a demolition expert. His temper could detonate over just about anything I did. Often when I least expected it. The shouting attacks started not long after we moved to our new one-bedroom apartment in West Los Angeles. Part of the reason behind his blowups was because he'd grown frustrated over the fact that I'd stopped cooking and cleaning regularly. But another part of the friction, I believe, came from Jerry's desire to be the greatest autistic leader on the planet. Back then he still had a lot of ego invested in AGUA—perhaps for good reason. With the formation of his support group, he'd finally pulled off something that was bigger than anyone—including himself—had dared dreamed. And now, I felt like he wanted to be reminded constantly of what a good job he'd done. He wanted praise, which is something everyone likes to hear. The problem was, I didn't particularly feel in the mood to keep heaping the compliments on him. And that's often when he lashed out the only way he knew—by yelling.

Once that happened, if I had the strength, I'd leave the apartment and go for a walk. But after a couple of months, a simple realization dawned on me. If nothing else, Jerry was a shouter. When he got mad that was how he expressed himself. He wasn't physically violent, but you wouldn't know that by listening to him. One night, not long after that little epiphany, something clicked inside me. Jerry had just returned from work and something about the fact that I hadn't stirred from bed all day set him off. Can't blame him, I suppose. But as he began shrieking at me, I suddenly felt myself crumple into a heap on top of the sheets. Before I knew what was happening, I'd curled myself up into a fetal ball, my hands cupped over my ears, rocking back and forth. Jerry's words bounced off me like pebbles. All I could hear was his muffled roar far off in the distance. Lying there the way I did, I'm sure I looked pathetic. But I was powerless to do anything about it. From that day onward, curling up into a lifeless lump seemed to be a perfectly natural response to Jerry's shouting. I was never quite sure how long I remained in that position, but inevitably when Jerry saw the effect his rage was having on me, he'd cool off and begin speaking in a normal voice.

When it came to marriage, I never paid enough attention to the interaction between my parents to learn how it worked. I realized that any marriage was filled with problems, but after a lifetime of setbacks and heartache, the headaches we were encountering quickly seemed insurmountable. Despite the domestic friction, there were moments when the bliss and the fairy-tale-like quality of our relationship would hang in the air so heavy I wanted to pinch myself out of fear that I might be dreaming. Whenever I felt strong enough, I'd try to have dinner ready for Jerry when he came home from work. The look on his face, the way it lit up when he smelled food bubbling on the stove, made me feel good about myself in a way I hadn't experienced in years. In spite of all the stress between us, I could tell he loved walking through the front door and finding his home filled with music, squawking birds, and another person who was happy to see him.

When I think back on those early days of our relationship, I realize that one of our problems stemmed from our feeling territorial about our talents. I could tell that my ability to paint was a frustration for Jerry. He had no clue where my ability came from or how I was able to summon it. I had a hunch I was channeling some creative force that was using me much like a computer uses a printer. It seemed beyond savantism. It was downright paranormal. After meeting Jerry, I began filling my canvases with numbers, creating numerical mosaics, which is something I'd never done before. I'd never allowed another person to influence my artwork. Yet whenever I showed a painting to him, he'd merely glance at it, then turn away. I'd attempt to point out that I was putting numbers in my paintings for him, but he was so sensitive about people seeing him as one of those one-trick ponies who could only crunch numbers that my creations only seemed to irk him.

The old wooden upright organ I'd moved into our place was another breeding ground for tension. Jerry would often sit down and amuse himself, picking out tunes by ear and, even though I enjoyed listening to what he created, I never had the wherewithal to compliment him enough. I now realize how much that must have hurt him. After all, he was attempting to share my interest in music, even though he was hardly a musical savant. Why I couldn't have offered up a few words of praise for him still pains me. Maybe it was because I harbored such a confused opinion of my artistic abilities? Then again, the real reason may have had more to do with my inability to hand out praise simply for the sake of being polite.

Jerry, however, appeared to enjoy listening to me play, especially a piece I wrote called *Horses,* which sounded a bit like a scaled-down symphony with a never-ending array of shifts in mood and meter. The problem was, I didn't enjoy performing for him because he suffered from the annoying "cocktail lounge syndrome." Instead of sitting there quietly and listening to me play, he'd talk and talk, making me feel like I was nothing more than a radio pumping out background music.

One evening, he announced that I played like an autistic. "You carry on quite smoothly for a while, then there's this inevitable break in the flow, followed by another long, smooth passage," he said.

I listened to Jerry's critique, then got up and went into the bedroom to think. His words didn't particularly strike me as an insult, but they did sting. When it came to my music, I didn't want to be autistic. I'd always imagined that my gift bypassed that part of my brain. I believed it came from another place, far, far away from that peculiar place that qualified me as an autistic.

Jerry and I both harbored a deep love for classical music. Although his knowledge of it was minimal, he was a sponge, ready to soak up anything I threw at him. My favorite opera was Mozart's *The Magic Flute,* which I'd once heard Beverly Sills's opera company perform at Lincoln Center. One night, when I popped a video of it into our VCR, Jerry's face lit up like a child at a video game arcade.

"I've always wanted to hear that," he gushed as we snuggled up together on the sofa.

This particular version of the opera opened with a man fainting after he spots a lizard jumping out of its hole in the ground. It was a funny-looking lizard, vaguely resembling an iguana covered with Christmas tree tinsel. The moment he saw it, Jerry roared with laughter, then grabbed the remote and reversed the scene, over and over again, so the lizard continually popped in and out of its hole. If I hadn't wrestled the remote out of Jerry's hand, we never would have finished watching the opera.

Which prompted me to say, "Jerry, you watch videos like an autistic."

"You're absolutely right," he replied, still roaring with laughter. "Now gimme that remote back."

Because I wanted my sons to see how happy Jerry could make me, I used to invite them over to our apartment for pizza and a movie. Steve, who had just started studying computer sciences at a vo-tech college in the area, was always happy to get a free meal. I have a hunch, however, that Jerry and I freaked the poor boy out when it came time to watch the night's chosen video, which usually turned out to be *Free Willy*. My eldest son has always been a stable, serious sort and was never quite comfortable when Jerry and I would "dress up" for movie night. I was still sporting my extreme crew cut at the time, so I particularly loved wearing my big white Mozart wig, along with a crimson leopard-print top and black leather pants. Jerry usually wore his killer whale costume.

There was nothing the two of us liked doing better than hamming it up during the movie, shouting out the characters' lines seconds before they actually spoke them. More often than not, Jerry would be "swimming" around the chairs and sofa in our front room, pretending to be Willy, a role he played perfectly. Jerry made a wonderful whale. He'd glide around the room so gracefully and with such clear focus. He rarely knocked anything over, although he did sometimes scare the birds a bit. And while all this was happening, Steve would just sit there, quietly chewing his pizza as our birds flapped around the room, their wings making the most wonderful whooshing sound.

"Here, Steve," I'd say, placing Shayna or one of our other feathered children on his head, "give your sister a bite of pepperoni pizza. She loves pizza."

Steve was always a good sport about that sort of thing. After all, he'd lived with me long enough to know that I always shared my food with my animals. But he'd been living on his own for a while by then, so sometimes I think he forgot what mealtimes were like at our house. So he'd nod politely, offer up an uneasy smile, and tear off a bit of cheese and crust for the animal that had just perched upon his head.

Due to my Asperger's-wired brain, I've always been a terrible mind reader—of mine as well as others'. But Steve was my son, so I always felt I knew exactly what the little voice between his ears was saying: Dear Lord, please don't let me turn out like this. And who could blame him? Certainly not me. And definitely not Jerry, who at that moment was usually swimming around in front of the TV in his homemade whale suit.

With Jerry and me, the good times were filled with a type of comfort and satisfaction that only we could relate to. They seemed heaven-sent. But the bad times, which often grew out of some insignificant slight or provocation, were intolerable. Perhaps other people might have been able to work through it all. But with us, the molehills quickly became big, ugly mountains with peaks enshrouded by dark clouds. We didn't dare scale them. In fact, just looking at them was painful. Sometimes, after Jerry would leave for work in the morning, I'd lie there under the sheets, staring up into the cottage cheese ceiling, and think about some disagreement we'd just had. I kept having these recurring thoughts that maybe all this—everything from my marriage to Jerry and my physical ailments—was some terrible dream. Like, maybe, I was actually lying in a bed in a nursing home somewhere, locked away in a coma, dreaming everything that had been happening to me over these past few years. That's the one thing I remember my sister Carolyn telling me about what happened to her during the months she spent in her coma. She'd imagined herself to be a frightened wolf wandering through a dark forest that was constantly changing and morphing from one strange thing to another. Could what was happening to me be any different? Any less hellish?

Some days, I'd lie there in bed, surrounded by our three baby iguanas, birds, and goldfish, and think about the way it had been, back when we'd first met, back when it was just the two of us and that was okay, because it was all we needed—just each other. But time had changed all that and so had my health. The doctors had run test after test, but they could never find the source of my sickness. Without the blessing of a name, I knew that deep down Jerry had begun to believe I was making everything up. Nothing could have been further from the truth. Losing my autonomy, watching my strength evaporate like water in the desert sands, was unbearable. I didn't want to hate Jerry, but I felt like I was suffocating.

The past few months had also reinforced the notion that I wasn't cut out to live in such close proximity to another adult. I'd spent years living with my sons, but they always seemed to have enough common sense to know when to give me some privacy. Maybe it was his Asperger's or maybe it was because he'd never been in a relationship before. Whatever the case, Jerry had yet to learn that precious skill of backing off. Perhaps he would one day. Then again, maybe he never would. All I knew was that if something didn't change soon, I would soon be pushed over the edge. And I knew myself well enough to understand that once that happened, all bets were off.

Thankfully, I could still paint and compose. At the time, my acrylic paintings had become bizarre visual puzzles based on people I'd known, all of whom were viewed from different, almost inhuman angles. Interspersed about the canvas were all sorts of symbols, numbers, and words. Sometimes one painting would join up with another one I'd paint weeks later. They were conundrums, multilayered maps depicting what I understood to be the strange terrain of reality that lay ahead of me, visual prophecies spelled out in a language that was both abstract and concrete, recorded in a language that only I understood. When I gripped it in my hand, the brush felt like it was being pulled by some invisible magnet. Every stroke was a surprise, yet purely automatic, like I was dancing over the canvas with my hands.

Not only did I create, but I destroyed, too. There were weeks when the only time I ventured outside our apartment was to douse my paintings with turpentine, then drop a match on them as they lay on the massive brick barbecue grill in the courtyard.

"Why are you doing this?" Jerry demanded to know on the evening he returned home from work to find me burning four of my canvases, which I'd spent the past three days covering with paint.

"I'm returning them to the universe." I laughed, mesmerized by the flames engulfing my creations. "The images will return to me eventually, only in another form." Even I could tell that Jerry thought I was nuts. I watched him run upstairs to our apartment to get a pot of water to douse my blaze. But by the time he returned, all that was left on the sidewalk was a pile of ash and charred wood.

The music I created often met the same fate as my paintings out on the sidewalk. I'd fill sheets of paper with my Bach-like creations, built upon the numbers two and three, all woven together to create what I felt were touchingly complex modulations of sound—at least they were touching to me. But who was I to judge? By that point I was taking so many medications that my nervous system had been reduced to a jumble of raw, deadened nerves that reacted in ways I could never quite predict. One afternoon, I found myself obsessed with the local news coverage of an RV that had gotten hopelessly wedged beneath a highway overpass. Before I knew it, that strange image from TV had driven me to compose a violin quartet, a languid, willow-like melody that sounded as if it had been created during the Elizabethan period. When I heard it playing inside my head, I began to sob. Which is exactly how Jerry found me when he walked in the front door.

He just stared at me, glancing periodically at the papers filled with my scrawled musical scores scattered around me on the floor. His silence made me nervous. I couldn't read moods, but I could often discern emotion from the sounds someone did or did not make. And at that moment, I could tell he didn't understand a thing about me. The way he saw it, I was just being lazy. Jerry supported my need to create, but he couldn't accept that I might possibly enjoy the sensation of allowing music or an image to flow through me onto the page without feeling the need to sell my creation to the highest bidder—providing there were any bidders at all. Besides, it just felt wrong to sell what I considered to be a gift from God. After awhile, I gave up trying to explain myself to him.

And he stopped asking me about it.

Despite all the craziness going on between us, the tension, misunderstanding, and frustration, the world Jerry and I dwelled in was insular and tiny. It was a universe populated by just the two of us. But when our story appeared on the cover of the *Los Angeles Times,* we'd become the hot new diagnosis of the moment. People couldn't get enough of our tale about how we'd found a way to love, thereby conquering the agonizing loneliness of autism. One day we were pariahs, the next we'd become the poster couple for this relatively little-known neurological condition known as Asperger's syndrome.

If only they knew how close Jerry and I were to tossing in the towel. Neither of us knew that there was more to love than just running around, going to the zoo, and acting silly together. It would be years before we learned that real, lasting love—the kind that can actually transform you—involves a lot of heavy lifting, a lot of hard work.

The days ticked onward, one flowing into the next in a way that no longer made sense to me. I lost track of time. I felt myself drifting away. For a while, it seemed like the only thing keeping me tethered to the here and now were my little projects that revolved around decorating our rental home. In fact, the one thing that Jerry and I did occasionally talk about was how nice it would be to use the proceeds from our pending movie deal to buy our rental house. The only catch was that during those chaotic times, I believed that if you went to the trouble of actually planning on something happening, it automatically meant that it was certain to happen. That being the case, I decided that since we *already* owned the house we were living in, it made perfect sense for me to paint a giant mural of Vincent van Gogh's *Irises* on the living room wall—all 8-by-20-feet of it.

Over a period of three months, I'd regularly bum a ride a couple of miles to an art supply store near our house and purchase as many tubes of acrylic paints and brushes as I could carry. I'd spend hours every day selecting colors, mixing them, then painting my giant mural upon my billboard-sized canvas. Even though I was reinterpreting the creation of another artist, the process of painting infused me with a sense of life I hadn't felt in some time. The more I painted, the more I felt an unshakable kinship with the tortured, misunderstood Vincent. God, what I would have done to meet him. No doubt the two of us would have hit it off. By all accounts, he created *Irises* in May 1889 after several episodes of self-mutilation and forced hospitalizations. He'd checked himself in to an asylum in Saint-Remy, France, and, in what proved to be the last year of his life, went to work creating almost 130 paintings. *Irises* was the first in this final explosion of creativity.

Some mornings, I'd stand there staring at the wall with some insipid TV game show cranked at full volume, while I pretended to be Vincent standing in the asylum gardens, zoning out on all those flowers as they swayed and twisted in the light wind. Those irises, the way they held themselves up on their vulnerable stems when the ground and the earth conspired to pull them back down, when all they yearned to do was ascend upward into the heavens— I knew that feeling so well. And the longer I contemplated that painting of his, the more I believed that Vincent's brain and mine shared a similar wiring.

I also knew this particular painting by heart, every pixel of it. So sometimes when Jerry and the boys came around, I'd tie a bandana over my forehead in the manner of a Japanese kamikaze pilot, so my eyes were blocked and I couldn't see a thing. And I'd continue painting, slowly feeling my way over the wall, pulled and directed by whatever that force was that had always been there for me for as long as I could remember whenever I picked up a brush or set out to compose music. As long as I got out of the way, it always did the rest. Blindfolded, all I saw was blackness. Yet I knew where every single curled, wavy brushstroke needed to go. I felt it with a certainty that was missing from every other aspect of my existence. If only I could have been guided by a similar force in my daily life.

Often, I'd be carrying on a conversation while doing all this painting, laughing, and carrying on, not paying a lick of attention to my creation, fully on autopilot. It was all a bit eerie for whoever might be watching—the notion that something so cohesive and whole could be produced by someone whose attention was constantly elsewhere. Maybe I was showing off a little bit. But why not? If you've got it, flaunt it—that's what I always say.

My home decorating projects didn't end with my wall mural. In fact, not long after completing my homage to Vincent's flowers, I decided to create a bit of living sculpture in the corner of the same room where I'd done all my painting. I just knew that our birds, iguanas, and rabbit desperately needed more nature in the house to be happy. My plan was simple, although backbreaking. One afternoon, I covered the carpet with plastic tarps and hauled in dozens of Easter baskets, which I'd transformed into planters filled with flowers and ferns.

"What are you doing?" Jerry screamed when he came home from work that night.

"It's a habitat for our children, Jerry," I informed him, in between trips to the backyard, where I dug up plants and requisitioned several large tree limbs for my project. "They don't have enough nature in their lives."

As much as he knew that creating a faux forest in a rental home (we never did buy it) might haunt us, Jerry knew I was right. Our scaled, feathered, and furry pets did deserve to be closer to Mother Nature.

On those days when I didn't have any strength and my anti-epileptic and pain medication had turned me into a vegetable, I'd sometimes think back to that strange, magical time when Jerry and I first met, back when we both felt like we'd hit the jackpot because we'd somehow managed to find someone so much like ourselves. Memories of those days would come drifting back to me in waves, one after another.

Once, while curled up under the dirty sheets of the makeshift bed I'd made from cushions on the living room floor, I caught a glimpse inside my head of the afternoon Jerry and I went on a walk during one of our first dates. For the first few minutes of our excursion, we entertained ourselves by trying to pronounce street signs backward. Then, for the simple reason that it seemed like a good idea, Jerry shouted: "The rule for today is that all buildings will wear sunglasses." For the rest of the day, every single building we encountered would be donning a pair of shades. I mean really, truly wearing a pair of enormous sunglasses.

I used to get a kick out of watching Jerry scrunch his face up on those rare occasions when the visualization mechanism inside his head temporarily went on the fritz and he was unable to glimpse the ridiculous image we'd both concocted in our heads.

"Gimme a minute," Jerry laughed, slapping the side of his head like one would a broken TV set. "It's just not coming to me."

Jerry had so much good in him. I didn't see it then, of course. I was too angry and too distracted by my physical pains. But every so often I'd catch small, fleeting glimpses of it. Sometimes when he was at work and my boys were out of the house, I'd creep into his room and pore through his poetry and other writings filling his journals. Despite his bizarre gift for numbers, he possessed an amazing sense of aesthetic. He truly was an artist, capable of experiencing the world on a much deeper level than I usually gave him credit for.

Not only that, but Jerry could spin the silliest, most whimsical stories on just about any animal or object he encountered. Or I should say, the old Jerry would do that, the one I'd fallen for way back when. The new Jerry, the one who'd taken the old one's place, was so uptight, so tightly wound and grumpy that he'd often stomp around the house angrily, whenever my sons and I were having a good time. I didn't know what to do with that Jerry, what to make of him. Maybe he was feeling the same way about me. All I knew was that I desperately wanted Jerry to lighten up, to enjoy the crazy ride we both found ourselves on. Why shouldn't he? Why shouldn't both of us? After a lifetime's worth of sadness and disappointments, why not milk our good fortune for everything we could?

I squeamishly put on a happy face when all those 60 *Minutes* cameras began following us. But I'm a horrible liar—unless, of course, I can somehow convince myself that I'm not lying. I suppose deep down a part of me still believed we could make it work. After all, I'd managed to survive all sorts of unpleasantness in my life. This was nothing, I told myself. In fact, the worse it got, the more I believed my unhappiness was forging me into a better person. Back then, I had this theory that personal suffering was the ultimate purifier, cleansing the soul, removing all impurities and traces of ego.

So when the 60 *Minutes* episode aired and I sat there with my sons and Jerry, I felt strangely uneasy watching the sappy spin they put on our relationship, convinced that everyone in the world must know we were trying to pull a fast one on them. Yet there was one thing that Jerry and I weren't lying about when those cameras began taping us for that *60 Minutes* segment. It was our chance to show millions of strangers that, although we might be weird, we certainly weren't useless or handicapped. It was clear by watching the segment that we possessed skills and talents that most people would be envious of.

The most surreal portion of the program came when one of the show's producers convinced some students at the prestigious Juilliard School of Music to play one of my modern compositions for strings. But instead of being blown away by the fact that one of my musical creations was being played by some of the nation's top musicians on prime-time network TV, I was annoyed. Their performance sounded so depressingly uninspired. It didn't take a musical savant to realize they'd only glanced at my music for a few moments before the cameras started rolling and were merely sight-reading it. Still, both my boys were thrilled to hear a musical composition penned by their nutty mother played on TV. They'd often heard me play some of my works on the piano, but to actually have a handful of respected musicians transform one from the abstract into the concrete was bewildering.

"I just don't understand how you do it," said Steve, shaking his head. "You go out of your way to write your music under the most awful conditions and it comes out sounding so . . . so beautiful. It's just weird, Mom."

My decision to kill myself came one month after my hysterectomy. The operation had done little to stop the excruciating, searing pains in my abdomen. Eventually, the doctors wrote me off as a hopeless hypochondriac and refused to run any additional tests. In fact, everyone from Jerry to our agent believed I was imagining the whole thing. And they both nearly burst a blood vessel upon learning that I'd had the audacity to telephone Steven Spielberg, demanding that he force my doctors to perform a series of radiological tests on me.

"You're going to ruin everything!" Jerry shrieked.

And that was when my troubled mind somehow convinced me that my husband was plotting to kill me, that I desperately needed to get away from him. So, on Christmas Eve, I planned my final escape. I wrote a letter to my boys, telling them not to cry for me, explaining why I'd chosen to end my life and how I wasn't quite sure if I'd be reborn into another body. Jerry popped his head in my door to say good night and I smiled at him. I pretended to be in a grand mood in order to prevent him from catching on to what I intended to do and spoiling my plans. Once he shut the door and the house grew quiet, I swallowed every pill I could locate in my bathroom—more than 250 painkillers and antiepileptics.

Then I lay down on my bed.

When I opened my eyes the next morning, a doctor was standing over me in the emergency room. He looked annoyed. "I can't quite figure out why you're still alive," he mumbled, shaking his head in disbelief. "At the very least, you're going to have liver damage."

Tears dripped down my cheeks. My sons didn't want to speak with me, they were so angry. Jerry looked at me and smiled, although I couldn't fathom what he could possibly be smiling about. What's a gal gotta do to get outta this life? I thought.

Six weeks later, I informed Jerry that I wanted a divorce. To hell with Hollywood and being a poster girl for autism, I wanted off the merry-go-round. Not long afterward, Peter and I shoved all our belongings into a U-Haul and headed east, out across the desert, back to the only place I'd ever considered home—Tucson. I wanted to clear my head and heal my body. I wanted freedom. The only problem is, I couldn't quite put a finger on what it was I wanted to be free from.

CHAPTER NINE

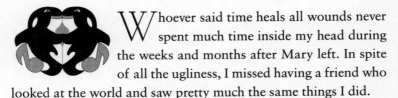Whoever said time heals all wounds never spent much time inside my head during the weeks and months after Mary left. In spite of all the ugliness, I missed having a friend who looked at the world and saw pretty much the same things I did.

Then, of course, there was *that* other reason. My ego just had too much invested in the two of us being Mr. and Mrs. Autism. All my life, I'd longed to be the center of attention, the focal point. Suddenly, I had half the heavies in Hollywood battling over me. It felt strange, but it was also wonderful to know that people were finally paying attention to Jerry Newport. I didn't want to let go of that feeling. So I racked my brain trying to understand why the universe would hand me this wonderful gift only to snatch it out of my hands before it came to pass. It wasn't fair. For weeks, I begged Mary to reconsider, to take me back, to keep the band together.

Despite my constant attempts at coping, I just couldn't shake Mary from my system. More than anything else, I missed the verbal connection we had. Mary truly gave great conversation.

She was intelligent, but in a truly unorthodox way. After a few painful months, as much as I hated to deny myself the temporary pleasure, I forced myself not to think about the good times we'd had together. It was just too painful. Then, one afternoon, just when I was about to hit rock bottom, I spotted a poster for a whale-watching class in Long Beach. I signed up for it and it soon became the one bright spot in my pathetic existence. The classes also rekindled my love affair with those massive beasts, reminding me exactly why I'd begun fixating on them in my childhood. The more I learned, the more I began to understand what we both had in common. Like me, a whale leads a predominantly lonely, isolated existence. But what I liked most about them was how they seemed so big, yet so full of grace. That was a quality I often wished I possessed instead of just feeling big.

After a year passed, I began embarking on the occasional date. And that was when I noticed something peculiar happening inside of me, something that made me think that maybe some scrap of good might come from all my heartache. That all-too-familiar sense of desperation I normally encountered when dealing with women had disappeared. I wasn't so quick to grasp at anyone who entered my life. I'd go out on a date with a woman and, when I admitted to myself that nothing was going to come of it, it didn't send the usual wave of panic through me. For a hopelessly insecure romantic like me, this feeling of control marked a true epiphany. For the first time in my life, I was the one who got to say, "There's no future in this," instead of being the one who had it said to him.

Another perk that came with having my heart broken was the sense of perspective it gave me. My fiftieth birthday was approaching and the more I pondered it, the more I had to admit how much happier I was than when I had turned forty. That was when my life truly seemed hopeless, shortly after my mother had died and I had no idea what I was going to do with my life. But now I told myself that, if nothing else, at least I'd finally done some living. In the past ten years, I'd had experiences I'd never dreamed possible. I'd managed to create a fuller, richer life for myself.

It was right around this same time that I was asked to speak at a fund-raising lunch for the Autism Society of Los Angeles. Instead of doing a variation on my usual this-is-my-wonderful-life speech, which I'd long ago grown bored giving, I decided to try something different. On a whim, I patterned my presentation on Gail Sheehy's bestselling book from the 1970s, *Passages*. I spoke about how those of us with autism experience passages in life, just like everyone else. Realizing you're different is a passage. So is finding your first friend, being ridiculed for the first time, leaving home, finishing school, getting your first job, and experiencing that awful first feeling of total hopelessness. Every human crosses those invisible lines of demarcation in life that lead us from one chapter to the next. Autistic people just do it in their own way, while traveling across terrain that is truly terra incognita to everyone but us. Every milestone in life is unique. So are the emotions that arise when we experience them. The important thing to remember is to just keep moving and try to enjoy the journey. Which is always much easier said than done.

Most of the time, I felt empty, like the only thing inside me was failure. It didn't take much time spent navel-gazing to realize that over the past twenty years, failing to measure up was the only thing I did with any real consistency. At least I'm good at that, I'd sometimes moan, doing my best to convince myself that I was nothing more than a washed-up math whiz, pot dealer, horse gambler, cabdriver, political campaign volunteer, bookstore cashier, and elementary school librarian.

Night after night, I'd lie in bed. The dull drone of accelerating traffic and people shouting in the street below would echo up into my apartment. I'd shut my eyes and watch as scenes and moments from my life flashed past my lids like some sloppily edited filmstrip. One image that I could never shake centered upon a memory of that hazy afternoon I learned that I'd landed an interview at the Occidental Petroleum Corporation in downtown Los Angeles. By then, I'd been out of the University of Michigan for a few years, long enough to sense my life was drifting into an uncontrollable slide, although the sensation still felt somewhat novel at the time. Months before, at the urging of my desperate mother, who I was living with at the time in her two-bedroom Santa Monica apartment, I set out to become an actuary, hoping to earn a living crunching statistics to calculate things like insurance premiums, risks, dividends, and annuity rates. If nothing else, it was a career that would allow me to put my mathematical skills to work. After passing two of the first ten rigorous licensing exams for actuaries, I found my way to Occidental and arrived there dressed in an old suit that I'd last worn to a fraternity social.

I didn't expect much. Why would I? I'd never received one significant job offer in my entire life that allowed me to make use of my freakish ability to crunch numbers. Why on earth would things change for me now? After I aced the company's in-house exam, a well-intentioned, fresh-faced human relations staff member took me on a walking tour of the company's neat and orderly offices.

With every step he took, he tossed another probing question at me. Even someone as socially dense as me could understand that every word he said was loaded. He was curious to know if I possessed any sense of direction, any inkling of where I wanted my actuary career to take me. It didn't take long for him to figure out that I was terminally clueless. At one point, as I attempted to answer his litany of questions, I summoned up enough courage to make eye contact with him.

I quickly wished I hadn't been so bold.

No sooner did I readjust my gaze from the floor to his face than I discovered he was rolling his eyes while listening to my answers. He smiled coolly upon noticing that I spotted him looking away, then walked me over to a giant oak door. He opened it just a bit and poked his head inside.

"Mr. Oldham," he announced in a very official tone, "this is Jerry Newport. He just passed the second phase of his national actuary exam and performed with flying colors on our in-house test."

The two men stared at each other quietly for a moment. Finally, Mr. Oldham nodded sternly, stood up, stretched out his hand, and said, "Hi, Jerry. I'm Ed Oldham, vice president of actuarial services at Occidental." All that separated us was his polished mahogany desk that appeared to be roughly the same size as a tennis court. He nodded at my interrogator, which I told myself must have been a cue for him to leave us alone and close the door behind him. I took a seat and jealously soaked in the plush, rich atmosphere of success that filled Ed Oldham's office. Sitting there in a perfectly tailored olive-colored suit, he launched into what I could tell was an oft-repeated oratory on the exciting career that awaits anyone who is accepted into the actuarial brotherhood at Occidental. He needn't have bothered; I was barely listening to a word he said. The view from his twentieth-story window of all the other high-rise office buildings, jutting up through a sea of custard-like smog, reeked of pure success, of arrival, of making it.

"So, Jerry," I heard him say, "what is it you like best about being an actuary?"

"The problems," I replied. "I like solving the statistical problems I'm given."

Mr. Ed Oldham nodded slowly, then frowned. This clearly wasn't the answer he wanted to hear. "Solving problems is all good and fine, but that's only part of being an actuary here at Occidental," he explained. "You need ambition, Jerry. Eventually, you have to make good decisions as an executive." He looked at me the way one might a plastic bag filled with garbage on a sidewalk. Even I could tell that he'd already formed a decision about me. Just as I'd predicted long before I showed up for this interview, I'd been judged unworthy. Part of me wanted to get up, walk out, and make this strange ritual of humiliation stop.

"So what is it you'd really want to do, Jerry?" he asked.

Having run out of the kind of energy required even to want to look into his eyes, I stared intently at the silver cup on his desk filled with pencils. "What I'd really like to do, I mean, if this interview is over, is go downstairs, get a hamburger at McDonald's, then take the bus out to Hollywood Park and bet on some horses."

"Oh" was the only word to come out of Mr. Ed Oldham's mouth. He promptly stood up, walked me out of his office, and down the hall to an awaiting elevator. "And thanks so much for stopping by, Jerry," he said, but even I could tell he didn't mean it. He walked back to his office, never bothering to turn around, even for an instant. Then the elevator doors shut.

Nothing quite like a trip down memory lane, I moaned every time I forced myself to relive that afternoon.

Night after night, images from my past came back to me in flashes—quick bursts of color and emotion that traced my journey from then to now, from nowhere to emptiness. Not long after that botched interview, I moved to San Diego, convinced that I could make my fortune using my math skills to make my fortune as a horse gambler. When that didn't pan out, I stuck around San Diego and became a cabdriver. Eventually, I ended up owning part of an independent taxi company, got my picture in the newspaper, and even ran for city council. But I soon made a mess out of everything and by 1985 I had lost my job, quickly run out of cash, and had no alternative but to return to my mother's apartment in Santa Monica. Because I didn't have enough money for a Greyhound bus ticket, I made the 135-mile journey with all my belongings stuffed in several trash bags, hopping from one city bus to the next. Despite the realization that my feat no doubt set some kind of weird public transportation record, I was horribly depressed by the time I arrived at the front door of my mother's apartment.

A few years and several dead-end jobs later, I got hired as a librarian at a nearby public elementary school. That moment marked a turning point in my life—and not just because it felt like I'd finally landed my first *real* job. It was there I touched my first autistic child, a lost little boy who, without knowing it, managed to reach out and plant a tiny seed inside my heart that took years to sprout.

One night while lying in bed with my forearm draped over my eyes, I caught a glimpse of him sitting in the back of the school library. It was in the second year of my job as the school librarian when I first laid eyes on ten-year-old Harrison, whose only form of communication in school was pinching the other kids. His fourth-grade teacher, at a loss over what to do with him, used to sit him down at a table in a distant corner of the library, put headphones over his ears, and let him listen to music. In between my duties shelving books or retrieving resource materials, I'd watch Harrison silently rock back and forth at his table. Although I couldn't quite put my finger on it, I felt a murky kinship with this uncommunicative little boy lost in a world nobody seemed able to penetrate.

Once, when his teacher spotted me watching him, she whispered, "He likes trucks."

"Trucks?" I asked.

"Yes, trucks," she replied. "His mother told me that he absolutely loves trucks."

When school let out that afternoon, I stayed in the library and found every book on the shelves containing a picture of a truck. After work on the way home, I purchased a half dozen toy trucks at a nearby drugstore. From then on, whenever Harrison would show up in the library, I'd arrange the vehicles in front of him on the table. He never lifted a finger to touch them, but he'd stare at the collection of big rigs until it was time to leave. Funny thing is, after a few months of watching him focus every shred of his attention on those toy trucks, I realized something no one else had.

"He's not really looking at the trucks," I informed his teacher. "It's the wheels that interest him. I think he must like circles."

"Circles?" she laughed. "What makes you think that?"

"I don't really know how to explain it," I said, thinking back to how I used to go out of my way to take taxi breaks at a Denny's parking lot filled with trucks. Something about watching all those wheels moving in unison calmed me better than any tranquilizer, although I didn't dare mention my pastime to Harrison's teacher. I told myself she wouldn't understand because I didn't understand why I did it or what was behind the peculiar effect it had on me.

Instead, I mentioned the record player. "Sometimes I let him watch records spin around on the turntable," I told her. "It seems like he calms down whenever I do that. After a few minutes of that, he seems far too happy to want to pinch anyone."

For the longest time, the nights were often the hardest part of no longer having Mary in my life. Almost like clockwork, around 9:30, the slide show inside my head continued—as did the deep funk I was powerless to pull myself out of. I couldn't shake the feeling that everything that had given meaning and joy to my life had begun to feel stale and pointless. I was growing too big for my past. Even my job, which had once seemed like a gift from the gods, was now doing nothing but frustrating and depressing me. After years spent working at UCLA, I'd begun butting heads with my boss. The tension started when I came up with a method I felt confident could help my department keep better track of the paper trail behind the myriad of purchases made by the university. Yet when I presented the idea to my higher-ups, it was ignored. Instead of trying to brainstorm ways to get my idea heard by the right person, I grew angry and frustrated, which I didn't bother to hide. Not long afterward, I began noticing that my duties were being constantly downgraded. Instead of spending my time auditing spreadsheets, I was asked to photocopy documents and deliver files to my coworkers. I retaliated by logging far too much time chatting on the phone and sending e-mails. My boss told me that I needed to focus more on my job, but I refused to listen. The lowest point came on the morning I arrived at my desk to discover that my computer had been taken away.

"You just can't take a hint, Jerry," my manager announced after I confronted her about the matter. She was right, of course. I'd always felt dense—especially when it came to interpreting and reacting to the delicate social world unfolding around me. But in the past at least I'd always attempted to do the right thing. At that point in my life, I just didn't care. It was as though the windows I gazed out of had become so smudged and dirty that I could only make out the shapes and outlines of what was happening outside. So I just gave up, pulled down the shades, and retreated into my own dark world. Why I never actually got fired still puzzles me. I certainly deserved it.

Even AGUA was beginning to frustrate me. I'd never expected to run the organization forever, but since no one in the group wanted to take it over, I was stuck with it. I needed to believe that it would outlive me, that years after I was dead this thing I created would be helping people. That meant a lot to me. But it didn't look like that was going to happen.

And ever since Mary's departure from my life, I couldn't shake the feeling that my passion for the group had gotten packed up in the back of that same U-Haul she'd taken to Arizona. Yet just when I felt like I wanted to toss the whole thing and be rid of it, I'd catch myself thinking about the way AGUA had actually made an impact in peoples' lives. And when that happened, I couldn't help thinking that perhaps my existence wasn't as meaningless as I'd been trying to make myself believe. If nothing else, our group was about possibilities. In its own subtle, unintentional way, it helped people visualize a future for themselves that perhaps they'd never imagined. All they needed to do was show up. The simple act of rubbing elbows with someone who actually had a real job, or a real girlfriend, or had moved out of their parents' house and was living on their own proved to be a powerful tool for transformation. It provided a sense of encouragement that went far beyond anything that most of our members had ever experienced. Someone in the group even compared it to being exposed to a virus: once this sense of limitless possibility got lodged inside your system, it was hard to shake. Over time, it mutated and replicated, eventually changing the way anyone exposed to it looked at their world.

For instance, the notion that someone could actually have a real career, instead of a throwaway minimum-wage job, proved to be a startling concept to just about all of us. But that's exactly what happened to one of our members named Ken, who had spent years sitting at home alone, drawing pictures on his computer. At one of our meetings, he happened to meet a father who had taught his autistic son how to create a variety of different types of art on his computer. It didn't take long for Ken to realize that he might be able to use his passion to actually earn a living, and he eventually became a graphic artist.

The notion that I'd played some small role in helping someone like Ken transform his life did wonders to lighten my blues. Exercise also improved my spirits. And after a few months spent hitting the weights and running on a treadmill at a fitness center near my apartment, I noticed I was sleeping better at night. Before long, the blackness began to lift just a bit. I tossed my bottle of antidepressants into the garbage. My appetite returned. Pretty soon, I began meeting people again and struck up a few friendships.

Then, one evening in October 1998, Mary telephoned and asked me to drive out to Arizona to pick up her birds. It was the first time I'd heard from her in more than a year. "I've run out of money," she explained, sounding tired and defeated. "I can't pay for their food this winter."

I didn't really want to see Mary. Visiting her was tantamount to playing Russian roulette with my brain. There was just no telling what sort of feelings it might stir up. Nevertheless, I agreed to help her. A few days later, I knocked on her door. She pulled it open slowly and we gave each other a quick, awkward hug. Mary resembled a zombie. I'd never seen her so listless and out of it.

We didn't say much to each other. I didn't realize it then, but she was submerged in the blackest depths of depression. It took me an hour to round up all nine of her birds—which she'd promised she'd have ready to go when I arrived—and place them in their cages. She muttered a feeble good-bye; then I traversed the five hundred miles back to my studio apartment in Venice Beach. A few hours after I left, Mary tried killing herself by once again emptying the contents of her medicine cabinet into her stomach. It didn't dawn on me until later that *this* was the real reason why she wanted me to pick up the birds: she didn't want them to be left alone. The realization that I'd been so oblivious to Mary's suffering only added to my own dark mood. I just couldn't believe I'd been unable to see it.

My own foul mood worsened. I was tired of everything about my life in Los Angeles and frustrated with my job at UCLA, where I'd been put on notice because of my dismal attendance. Then one night, a few months after Mary's botched attempt at ending her life, I also tried committing suicide by swallowing what I'd imagined would be an overdose of sleeping pills. The only thing that happened was that I realized that perhaps living wasn't such a bad idea after all. Not long afterward, while traveling for one of my out-of-town speaking gigs, I started thinking: Why not move? Why not pull up stakes and leave Los Angeles, where a person has to earn $2,000 a month just to be poor? But whenever I thought about moving, all I thought about was that I made too much money at my stupid job ever to have the guts to leave.

Then, once again, my telephone rang. It was Mary. I hadn't heard from her since our last dismal attempt at getting back together months before. As much as I didn't believe it, she actually sounded sane for the first time in years. When I happened to mention how tired I was of living in Los Angeles, she said I ought to think about moving to Tucson.

"It's cheaper out here," she said. "We could give it another try. No strings attached."

I was skeptical, but I still missed Mary. Yes, I'd moved on, but

I never felt complete without her. So a few weeks after that conversation, I drove out for a visit. Not long afterward, Mary came to see me. Although I forced myself to be cautious and take things slowly, she actually seemed like a new woman—or maybe just the old one I remembered from back when we first met. My friends told me I was crazy even to consider getting back together with her. But they also admitted that my getting out of Los Angeles might not be such a bad idea. One afternoon, I spotted Bert, an old cabbie buddy from San Diego I hadn't seen in more than a decade. He was hobbling down a sidewalk in Venice Beach, clutching a cane. I desperately needed someone like Bert to talk to. So, before I even realized what was happening, I blurted out that I was thinking about getting back together with my ex-wife. Bert listened, then shook his head and grinned.

"Sometimes," he chuckled, "you need another shot—just so you can know if you want to keep sipping from that same bottle or if you should heave it in the trash." I took that to mean that he was in favor of my move.

I had no idea what it was I was looking for on that afternoon in March 2001, when I stuffed all my belongings into my beat-up blue Mazda, complete with personalized IMDAWHL license plates, and struck out toward Arizona. What I did know was that this time around things would be different. I knew all her tricks, I told myself.

This time around, I wasn't going to let her break my heart.

TUCSON, ARIZONA
MAY 1997

Here's how my new life without Jerry began. My thinking may have been clouded, but I knew one thing: I desperately wanted a permanent home for me and my animals. Persuading someone that a person in my mixed-up state of mind could be trusted to pay a mortgage wasn't easy. But I finally located a run-down house in a dusty barrio on the fringes of Tucson that cost only $65,000. Between what little money I still possessed, some help from Ron Bass, the screenwriter of our movie, and even Jerry, I put down $20,000. I showed the seller a copy of our contract from Dream-Works, promising me more money for several years, easily enough to live on and make payments. I was so desperate that I accepted a variable-interest-rate loan on the remaining portion, which eventually climbed to an astronomical 13.75 percent.

A few days after moving in, I stood in my new backyard, which was nothing more than a stretch of hard-packed dirt and sand, and experienced a revelation.

"This house needs a grave!" I shouted.

Before long, I'd located an old garden trowel, a hammer, and a screwdriver in one of my closets, then calmly walked outside and began scraping a hole in the concrete-like ground. I kept at it for the next six hours. Days and weeks passed and I kept scraping, retrieving artifacts out of my ever-widening hole, everything from chicken bones and a few assorted cat skulls to decades-old trash.

Despite the good time I was having digging, I'd never felt more alone in my life. My parents, who had moved to California years before, had refused to speak to me and had once again cut me off. My insides still ached from my hysterectomy and the diverticulitus that made my intestines throb and burn. To make matters worse, even my HMO had given me the boot.

And still I scraped my hole in the ground. Every day, my neighbors, most of whom were Mexican immigrants, walked past my property on their way to work at the nearby bottling plant or brickyard. They stared at me, blank expressions on their smooth brown faces, absolutely perplexed by what their crazy gringo neighbor was doing. None of them read English, but I'd hung signs on the fence in front of my house anyway: MY HMO IS KILLING ME! The banner certainly made sense to me. Eight months earlier I'd phoned DreamWorks, demanding that the famous director and producer find me a specialist who could cure me. I never heard back from him, so it only seemed natural to blame him for all my physical woes.

"That's why I'm digging my grave!" I'd shout to the passersby. "I'm dying!" After awhile, they began to smile and wave.

Some days I couldn't summon up enough energy to drag myself out of bed. The pains inside me had subsided just enough to make life tolerable, but all the digging I'd been doing brought the agony back with a vengeance. Yet whenever I could stand the discomfort, I continued cutting into the earth. One afternoon, about five feet down, I struck an ash-white layer of limestone. I poured bucket after bucket of water into my grave and spent the better part of several days soaking my body in the milky liquid. The alkaline content of my makeshift bathwater soothed the lesions covering my skin, and they soon disappeared.

I started painting again and composing my music. My property was covered with prickly pear cactuses. Since money was running so low, I'd begun picking the edible pads off the plants and cooking them with a blowtorch. The pads, known to my Mexican neighbors as *nopalito,* tasted a bit like squash and were packed full with vitamins and amino acids. One day I asked several of the barrio kids, all of whom were Yaqui Indians, to dip their bare feet in red paint and march around my house. A few of them lay on my floor and I outlined their bodies in red and white paint. I enjoyed referring to the images they left behind as death angels.

My life was proceeding along crazily but fairly predictably and then it happened. One afternoon, I dragged myself out of bed, opened the front door, and watched in horror as a band of black helicopters raced past overhead. Something about that vision, something about that guttural thumping sound of the rotors unleashed a terrible horror inside me. I didn't know then what it was, but I've come to understand that those choppers stirred up a dark, ugly memory that I'd spent almost two decades trying to forget. The nearly deafening noise forced me to relive the terrible months my boys and I were held prisoner by a deranged, shell-shocked Vietnam vet named Lars. In a life filled with so many ugly, traumatic events, my time spent as his psychological hostage proved to be the most devastating. Whatever was wrong with the wiring inside my head before meeting Lars was minor league stuff compared to the permanent mess he made of my neural circuitry. He transformed me from a loopy hippie chick with Asperger's into an often paranoid shut-in convinced that the world was out to get me.

When we first met in 1979, Lars was a neighbor in Tucson. He moved into my rented house and took control of my life. In the months that followed, he beat my sons, led us on forced marches through the desert with barely any water, threatening to murder us so many times that the terror of his words almost began to feel normal. As kidnappers go, Lars was pure genius. He found the perfect victim: me. Like a lot of people with Asperger's, I take things literally. And Lars soon learned that this was his ultimate weapon against me. His detailed threats about what he was going to do if I ever tried to escape kept me hostage far more effectively than if he'd merely chained me up and placed a gag in my mouth. Even worse, he sensed that I didn't care much about protecting myself, yet I harbored a fanatical need to protect the handful of people I loved. So that was who Lars went after—my boys and my parents.

"You even think about leaving and here's what I'll do," he'd seethe. "First, I'll set fire to your parents' house, then I'll wait outside with a rifle and blast them to smithereens when they try to flee. It'll be just like shooting mice in a bucket."

Lars also understood that since I had the reputation of being something of a kooky eccentric in the community, the police would never believe me when I went to them with my wild claims that my boys and I had been abducted. Like the afternoon when Lars went out to score some Valium and I finally summoned enough courage to phone the cops.

"You've got to help us," I whispered into the receiver. "He keeps saying he's going to kill us."

"How long has he been telling you this?" the desk sergeant asked, already sounding a bit skeptical.

"For the past six months," I whispered. "It started not long after he abducted us."

"Lady," the officer explained, "if he was gonna kill you, he would have done it by now."

End of conversation. He hung up the phone. The authorities wrote the whole thing off as an ugly case of boyfriend-girlfriend love gone bad. Even my parents were convinced that I was somehow to blame for the whole mess. So when it was all over, when Lars finally got tossed in jail (he skipped town the moment he was released, weeks before going to trial), I gathered up all those horrible memories and all the shame of not being able to protect my sons, and crammed all that hurt inside a tiny box that I locked away deep inside my heart. The only problem was the lock never seemed to work and the contents of the box occasionally spilled out. Whenever that happened and the horrible memories became too vivid, I'd get carted off and locked away inside a mental institution, which wasn't as bad as it sounds. Besides meeting some truly delightful people, one of the perks of getting sent to a mental institution was that I inadvertently learned what it felt like to be firmly rooted in the here and now—a sensation that's a completely alien experience for someone whose brain is hardwired the way mine is.

It happened on the morning of my first day, after I challenged some orderlies who I believed were roughing up an elderly "guest" at their facility. I was tackled, wrestled down to the linoleum, and dog-piled by several hundred pounds' worth of burly guards. The sensation felt similar to being hit by a city bus. I enjoyed it immensely. It was strangely . . . *comforting*. Having all that mass piled on top of me, flattening and squeezing me down into the linoleum suddenly allowed me to feel the outlines of my physical body perfectly defined and delineated. For the first time in my life, I knew exactly where I was. The fuzziness of my existence vanished and was momentarily replaced by one of sharp, defined focus. It felt like I was flying.

Here's something else I learned from my stays in various mental hospitals: contrary to what most people are led to believe, the hallways of most state institutions are not crawling with psychiatrists, psychologists, and therapists. In fact, I rarely encountered any. Occasionally, I was allowed to speak with a staff therapist. Not that those visits ever brought me any lucidity. In fact, whenever I brought up the part about how Steven Spielberg had bought the movie rights to my life story, my therapist would furrow his or her brow and tell me: "Now, Mary, we both know that's not true. Don't we? We both know that nobody is making a movie about your life. Don't we?"

"But—" I'd protest.

"Now, Mary," they'd reply. "Why don't we just stop all this nonsense?"

After awhile, I just gave up trying to convince them. Why bother? In fact, the more I thought about it, the more I had to admit that the whole thing sounded pretty crazy. Eventually, I began to suspect they were right. After all, why would anyone want to make a movie about me?

In between getting pumped full of medication to drive the delusions out of my head, I spent a lot of time during my stays at those various institutions thinking about my life, scanning the horizon behind me for proof that I hadn't always been such a hopeless mess. Like that time after all the dust settled from the Lars fiasco, when I followed my gut and everything actually worked out.

It all started when my son Peter's first-grade teacher insisted that I should place him in a special-ed class where he could work with a speech pathologist. Although he was already six years old, his entire vocabulary consisted of a handful of consonants. Whenever he did attempt to speak, he'd blow air through his nose and grunt. If I hadn't been his mother, I would have believed him to be feral.

"It's okay," I'd tell him. "There are other ways to communicate besides words. When you're ready to start talking, it'll happen. There's no rush."

When I thought about what the specialists told me, I had serious doubts he'd ever learn to speak. Yet, deep down in that place where I stored all my optimism, I knew the words would eventually rise up to the surface and float off his lips. He just needed someone who believed in him, someone who could be patient and wait him out.

Peter's speech therapy classes only made things worse. After his sessions, he'd come home so stressed and flustered that he sounded like Porky Pig. So one day I just stopped taking Peter and his brother to school and set out to find a way to help him. Not long afterward, it dawned on me that since Peter had always been attracted to music, maybe that was where the answer lay. Although no one could really understand him, he loved to sing.

And that was when the neon light turned on above my head. "Don't focus on the words," I told him one morning after he crawled out of bed. "Just listen to what people are saying as though it were music, then try to create your words like you would sing a song."

When I first suggested that to him, Peter stared at me and smiled faintly, but not so faintly that I couldn't understand he was smiling. Whenever we'd go somewhere in the car, I'd roll down the windows instead of turning on the air conditioner, and we'd listen to the blasts of air billowing in, colliding with our faces. We did a lot of listening during those next few months, paying attention to sound, trying to understand the melodies in everything from a windstorm to a boiling tea kettle. Peter couldn't have asked for a better cohort during this process. After spending so much of my life feeling different from everybody else, feeling as though I were sealed off from the rest of the world by some impenetrable force field, I told myself I knew exactly what he was going through. All I could offer him was patience and empathy because that was really all that I possessed.

Nothing happened for a while. Not even someone with my acute, freakishly sensitive hearing could detect any discernible differences in Peter's speech. But he was smiling more and I could sense he felt more relaxed, which meant everything to me. Then one morning, months later, it happened. He plodded into the kitchen in his pajamas, rubbing the sleep from his eyes. A perfectly enunciated, crisp "Hi, Mom" fluttered out of his mouth before he sat down at the table, giving me his trademark where's-my-breakfast stare. Although I wanted to jump up and down and start dancing, I knew the last thing he needed was for me to make a big deal out of the fact that he'd finally learned to speak.

Instead, I roughed up his hair, poured him a glass of orange juice, and asked, "You want waffles or pancakes?"

One afternoon while killing time in the rec center of a nameless facility outside of Tucson, I found myself thinking back to my days when I worked as an itinerant piano tuner, a vocation that finally allowed me to put my uncanny hearing to good use. I learned the bulk of my trade in Los Angeles during the mid-1980s, after landing a job with one of the city's top piano rental firms. I worked hard, harder than I ever had at anything in my life. But with ears as delicate as mine (my boss once described them as "wolf-like" because of their ability to hear sounds others couldn't), I was a quick study. Most tuners I knew required about two hours to fully bring a wayward piano back into tune. Using an electronic scope, it took me just forty-five minutes.

Before long, I was traveling around Southern California, tuning pianos for folks such as Herbie Hancock, Burt Bacharach, Crystal Gayle, and Don Henley. For the first time in my life, it felt like I was punching a hole through the barrier that had surrounded me for decades. I began to view myself as something more than just a talented amateur. As strange and unlikely as it seemed, I felt on the verge of becoming a professional. Surely it was only a matter of time before I'd laid enough of a foundation and paid enough of my dues to pursue my secret dream—composing music that people would take seriously.

Eventually, the boys and I moved to Manhattan and I found my skills in demand. I was soon working in such places as the Apollo Theatre and Radio City Music Hall. I tuned for Broadway shows, classical radio stations, recording studios, restaurants, and lounges. I even made house calls—at least until I encountered one too many apartments filled with shrieking children and television sets cranked up to full volume. On more than one occasion, in some stranger's apartment, I nearly experienced a full meltdown due to the overload of noise. It felt like a railroad spike was being hammered through my head.

Sometimes, when I look back over that period, I think my ears got too sensitive from all the tuning I was doing, too intolerant of sonic discord. Not long afterward, I crashed and burned. Because of my reputation as a talented yet highly unstable crank, nobody wanted to hire me anymore.

I don't really miss the profession. But I've always wished I could find someone who could bring me back in tune.

The story behind my reunion with Jerry a year later went like this: I was flat broke. My mortgage hadn't been paid in months. On any given day when I returned home from my shift at the sandwich shop, I expected to find my front door chained shut and all my possessions piled in a Dumpster. Much of my time was spent fantasizing about the day I'd finally be forced to begin living and sleeping in an appliance box on the dusty streets of Tucson. Actually, the prospect didn't really depress me that much. And after awhile, it actually began to excite me a bit. It began to feel like yet another wild, inevitable adventure, the natural next chapter in the long, drawn-out story of my life. So, one day before I figured my telephone would be turned off, I dialed Jerry's number. I'd been thinking about him a lot lately. And each time a memory popped into my head, all the good things about Jerry started coming back to me—things I hadn't thought about in years, tiny snippets of moments that tugged the corners of my lips into a smile.

"Hi, Jerry," I said, when I heard his voice on the other end of the line. He didn't really seem surprised to hear from me. But he did sound suspicious, even a bit regretful that he'd answered the phone. I told him everything I'd been thinking about over the past few months. I told him about my situation with the house.

Something about his monotone, somewhat emotionless voice sounded vaguely *down*. What was wrong? I asked. He reluctantly told me how burned out he was from living in Los Angeles. He wanted a change in his life. So I hit him with my offer.

"We both know you wanted things to turn out differently between us," I told him. "I think I do, too. Lately, I can't just help wondering what might have happened with us."

Jerry stayed quiet for a moment. "What's the catch, Mary?" he asked suspiciously.

"Move out here," I told him. "Live with me and I'll turn the house over to you. You'll own it."

"And?" he grumbled. He'd embarked on far too many of my roller-coaster rides to allow himself to get excited over anything I might tell him.

"And I'll be the most hardworking, stable wife a man could ever want," I replied. "You'll see. And if things don't work out, then at least we'll know we gave it our best shot."

Jerry got quiet again. All I could hear was the sound of his breathing traveling over hundreds of miles of phone lines.

"Jerry," I finally asked. "You still there?"

"I'm thinking," he replied. "I'm thinking."

CHAPTER TEN

TUCSON, ARIZONA
APRIL 2001

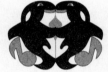The curtain for my second act with Mary had barely gone up when it hit me—Mary had a lot in common with an old radio I once owned. When her signal was coming in loud and clear, I could sit there listening to her carry on all night long, truly awestruck by the beauty and magic of what I was hearing. Yet, if her dial accidentally got nudged or bumped, even just a smidgen, the music ceased and all I heard was an earful of discordant static. There was definitely plenty of beautiful music in those early days after we decided to give our relationship a second go. The two of us were getting to know each other all over again. Only this time around, we were both a bit wiser to all the tricks our heads, our hearts, and our brains wanted to play on us.

In those opening moments of Jerry and Mary, Part II, I was in a good place. Finally pulling myself out of the chaos of Los Angeles did wonders to calm my head. It felt as though a weight had been lifted from my shoulders. Not long after arriving, I went to work creating an Asperger's support group for adults in Tucson. We held our first meeting at the sub and pizza shop where Mary worked in the kitchen as a cook. During those first few meetings while everyone became comfortable with one another, I'd snatch glances at her back by the ovens, watching her juggle a dozen different orders at once, additional ones being tossed at her every few minutes. The sight was absolutely mind-boggling. I'd never known anyone with Asperger's who could multitask like that, who could handle all that overload of variables and uncertainties, yet somehow not lose it. For the first time since we'd met, Mary was running on all eight cylinders, more focused and driven than I'd ever seen her. She was also working herself ragged, which wasn't necessarily a bad thing.

With Mary bringing home the bacon, I finally enjoyed the privilege of staying home and trying my hand at writing the book I'd been putting off for years. Ever since our 60 *Minutes* spot aired, publishers had been approaching me to publish my biography. The last thing I wanted to do, however, was spend any more time dwelling on my oft-told story. I'd grown tired of it. Yet ever since moving to Arizona I'd decided to get really serious about finding a way to use what I'd learned from life to try to help others in the autistic community. So I decided to create a self-help book, signed a deal with a publisher, and went to work pounding away on my keyboard, day and night for several months. And when *Your Life Is Not a Label* finally came out in September 2001, I'd often sell it after my speeches. The best part was when people would ask me to pen something inside the copy they'd just purchased. At first I never quite knew what to write. Then it hit me: why not put my number-crunching prowess to work? Before long, I was asking anybody who bought a copy the same question: "When were you born?" The moment they told me, I'd go to work calculating how many days old they were, then scribble the number above my signature. Everyone always got a kick out of that.

❧

The only downside to my new career as an author was the size of my royalty checks. For some reason, I'd fantasized that more digits would be involved, especially since Mary's job just barely covered our mortgage, utilities, and the bit of food we kept in the kitchen. I'll never forget that afternoon when I excitedly ripped open the envelope that had just arrived in the mail from my book publisher. All I could do was laugh when I saw the size of the check inside.

"What are we gonna live off of?" I groaned. Mary glanced down at the piece of paper clutched in my hands and giggled.

"I've got an idea," she announced, opening the front door and pointing down the street. "Why don't you take a look down there?"

Curious as to what she was talking about, I walked outside and squinted in the bright sunlight, trying to make out the wording on a sign bolted into a nearby brick building.

"Oh!" I laughed, dumbfounded by what I saw. "I guess I never noticed that before."

Sure enough, at the end of the block was a cab company. I pulled on my sneakers and wandered down the street to investigate. They hired me on the spot. As much as I swore I'd never work as a cabbie again, it didn't take long to realize I was enjoying my old job in a way I never had before. It felt nice to be back behind the wheel of a taxi again, more comfortable than I ever remembered it could be. At first I couldn't put my finger on it, but after a few months the answer came to me. Back during my years spent driving in San Diego, I'd always been embarrassed by the fact that I was forced to pilot a cab in order to pay my rent. Not a day went by when I didn't worry what people must be thinking when they climbed inside my vehicle and told me where they wanted to go. Surely just one glance at the back of my head was all it took before they sensed what an awful disappointment I was, how I'd failed to live up to all the hype and promise that had been heaped upon me while growing up.

But this time around, I didn't feel like a loser. Why? Because

I'd managed to acquire a past I could look back on and be proud of. Whenever I felt the least bit down, I could tell myself that I'd done something with my life and actually believe it. That made all the difference. So, if driving a cab was what I wanted to do to help myself buy my daily whole wheat bread, then I'd do it my way and not feel I had to apologize to anyone.

The longer I careened through the sweltering, dusty streets of Tucson while piloting my taxi, the more I began to sense subtle shifts occurring deep inside me. The sensation was similar to the seismic tremors that used to shake the ground in Los Angeles when I lived there. Thanks to technology, my job was easier and less stressful than it had been back when I was driving cabs in the 1970s. All the information I needed now appeared on a computer screen mounted on my dashboard—where my fares would be waiting, destination information, and so on. That meant I rarely had to scream into my radio at a dispatcher, an activity that always sent me into a crabby funk. Tucson was also a much more pleasant place to drive than San Diego or Los Angeles—no ugly intersections anywhere, always a mountain or something nice to fix my eyes upon, no matter where I stopped. Not as much traffic, either. The pace suited me perfectly.

All I had to do was drive, which gave me time to think, to try to ponder where I'd come from and where I was going. Rarely a day went by when I didn't experience some slight glimmer of insight into what made me tick. The first epiphany centered on my mortality. For the first time, instead of telling myself that the bulk of my life lay ahead of me, I had to admit that just the opposite was true. This led to another realization: most of the little things I'd spent so much energy dwelling upon just weren't worth worrying about. So what if I hit one red light after another? What can I really do about the traffic jam on the way to the airport?

As strange as it sounds, driving a cab became something of a meditation for me. And for the first time in my life, I was enjoying an activity with no strings attached. Just being able to provide a service for another human, to transport him from point A to point B, felt so positively blissful that I wondered how I'd managed to ignore it for all these years. All my disappointments over the past or freak-outs over what might or might not happen in the future no longer worried me. I was plugged into the present moment in a way I never had been before. The more I drove, the more I began to sense things about myself that had always remained hidden.

One afternoon, a few hours into my shift, I realized how my entire life had been held hostage by my overblown sense of inferiority. The epiphany nearly floored me. In the blink of an eye, all the chatter inside my head, all those mean-spirited voices that constantly browbeat me into believing that everything I did was never enough, went mute. They'd finally run out of wind or perhaps they just realized I wasn't listening anymore. And in their place came a serene, comfortable quiet.

No matter how hard I tried, I couldn't shake the feeling that it was Mary who had helped me finally locate the volume knob. My years spent with her had given me the space my heart and mind needed to make peace with each other. From what I knew about its powers, love isn't what does the healing. Love simply lays the necessary groundwork so that we can do the healing ourselves. This realization left a bittersweet taste in my mouth. After all, I was fifty-one years old. The fact that both my father and grandfather had died of heart attacks at the age of sixty-one meant that I might have less than ten years to live, which forced me to look back over my life with a sense of clarity I never knew I possessed. For once, instead of getting depressed over what I saw, I felt the stirrings of something resembling satisfaction. I may not have gotten everything I wanted out of life, but—to paraphrase Mick Jagger—I got what I needed. And for the first time, I was okay with that.

Despite all my insecurities and self-flagellation, I concluded that my life had actually amounted to something. I'd forged my own path. That was important to me. Maybe it came from all those episodes of *The Untouchables* I watched as a kid. But I just liked the idea of being the type of person who couldn't be bought off. I was an untouchable not because of my aversion to physical contact, but because I stuck to my guns and clung to what my gut told me was right. The close-minded, antiquated ideas of others couldn't touch me. Of course, this brashness didn't particularly endear me to everyone in the autism community.

Back in 1993, lots of folks believed that the idea of an autistic-adults-run support group for autistics bordered on lunacy. But they were wrong. And today there are at least a couple dozen support groups, all based on the AGUA model, thriving around the nation. But back in those dark ages, a few well-meaning, hopelessly ignorant souls believed that packing too many autistics together in one place might actually make our condition worse—as if our neurological disorder were contagious and might rub off on those of us only predisposed to it. Others insisted that we wouldn't be capable of undertaking such a gargantuan, unprecedented task without supervision. At the very least, we'd need to hire a "professional" to oversee it.

Since moving to Arizona I was still involved with AGUA, but I'd drifted away from the actual group. No longer was it the central focus of my life. Yet it was an indelible part of me. Mary had her two sons, who have both grown into fine young men. I had AGUA, which had grown in its own unique way. And it was time for me to begin allowing it to stand on its two legs, to see if it was strong enough to make its own way in the world without my constant attention.

Still, I wonder about so many of the people whose paths intersected mine back when AGUA was such an integral part of my existence. I think about all the mothers who encouraged and supported me when I started it. And I think about their sons, the ones they were so desperate to help lead more normal lives, to help them have any lives at all. Sometimes, at the strangest moments, I catch myself wondering how many of these sons—or daughters— have managed to gain the friends and independence their moms so badly wanted them to make through the group.

I know Ilene Arenberg did. She was an original member of AGUA who now works as a full-time employee of UCLA, lives in her own apartment, and takes the bus to work every day. Clearly, Ilene's progress has been influenced by all the people she met through AGUA who expanded her view of what was possible in life. In my book, she's definitely a success and a heroine. But not just because of her vocational progress. Ilene has managed to mature into a wonderfully adjusted adult while still being a person who is undeniably autistic.

And then there's Derrick Hall. He pops into my mind from time to time, and the memory of him never fails to make me smile. Growing up, Derrick never knew he had autism. He had no idea why he took all that medication or ended up in classes separate from the other kids at school. It wasn't until his late twenties and he'd lost his job at the post office that his mother finally broke the news to him.

"Man, was I shocked," he told me a couple of years later. Despite the pain of his hurt, he ranks as one of the most courteous, sensitive, fair-minded humans I've ever had the privilege of meeting. He's a handsome, fit man, who has a healthy marriage that came later in life. More than anything since my move to Arizona it's Derrick's infectious outlook on life that I miss most. I couldn't stand next to him without feeling the incandescent glow of his spirit. He's living proof that an autistic person can grow up and learn to appreciate the forest as well as the trees.

Jessica is another AGUA member who all I have to do is think about and I suddenly feel as though I've been enveloped by a cloud of sweet-smelling perfume. Her personality has grown and evolved so much over the years that I've known her. Jessica ended up in an institution when young and was rescued through adoption. After learning about our group, she took a long time to relax and realize that hanging out with "a bunch of autistic nuts" like us wouldn't threaten her security. But eventually she began referring to us as friends. She's the type of person who is literally consumed by her interests (she loves airplanes and making sketches of buses). Watching her face light up when she spots a jet flying overhead is a sight you don't easily forget. Now in her late forties, she's vintage autism at its best, and a person not nearly as alone as she once was, thanks to AGUA.

And then there's Sharon. She burst into our scene like a hand grenade in 1994, shortly after moving to LA from New York. She scared the living hell out of me during that first meeting she attended. Our little group apparently didn't quite measure up to what she'd envisioned for a support group and she felt no qualms about telling me just how displeased she was. Good lord, what a kindred spirit! We laughed about it years later while having lunch at the Getty Museum, during an AGUA group trip there. Sharon recently moved to the desert, outside of Los Angeles, thanks to Hal, another member who befriended her and tirelessly worked to help her deal with issues like aging and retiring.

Hal and his buddy, John, are the true world travelers of AGUA. They both get a kick out of attending autism conferences in various parts of the country and regularly travel to Autreat, an annual retreat held on the East Coast, sponsored by Autism Network International. Hal spent years working with the city of Los Angeles's planning department and took an early retirement. John loves doing volunteer work all over the world for his church. It's too bad they're both on the road so much. Looking back on those early days, I didn't know what to make of either of them when they both arrived at our meeting. None of us did. They both seemed to cope so well with so many of the things that tended to push most of us over the edge. There were plenty of days I wondered if they really belonged with us. But eventually, they passed our "autism test"—although I've never quite figured out what exactly that is. I guess all of us just decided that if those two guys were crazy enough to want to spend time with us, they must be like us.

The more time I logged behind the wheel of my cab, the clearer my head became. I began looking at myself in a way I never had before. I actually started to believe the heretical notion that I'd accomplished something with my life. But the funny thing is, I'd probably still be beating myself up if I hadn't let Mary drag me out to Arizona, where I got to experience more space and quiet than I ever had in my life. If anything had allowed the flower within me to blossom, it was Mary. (Not to mention all the manure I'd dumped on myself over the course of my lifetime.)

One afternoon while shuttling a harried businesswoman to the Tucson International Airport, I experienced a flashback, a split-second vision of myself standing in the showers after gym class while a group of guys snickered at my anatomy. The memory made me cringe. I wanted to pull my cab over to the side of the highway and start screaming at those idiots who had somehow hoodwinked me into hating myself. But I didn't. Instead, I just kept on driving while fighting back a torrent of tears threatening to burst loose from my eyes. After a few minutes, I heard myself whisper, "Forget about it, Jerry. That was years ago. You gotta let go of all that now. You have to forgive them. They certainly wouldn't have laughed at you if they'd thought you were going to keep dwelling on it for nearly forty years. It's time to move on." So that was exactly what I did. I punched the gas and moved on down the highway, making it to the airport in record time.

"Wow!" My fare laughed as I screeched to a stop beside the curb. "That didn't take long."

"Only about four decades." I chuckled as I climbed out of the car to fetch her suitcase from the trunk.

Not long after that trip, I began to make a conscious effort to incorporate all the epiphanies I was experiencing into my daily life. More than anything, I yearned to use them as a tool to help me cobble together a bit of sanity whenever I encountered one of those moments that normally tended to push me over the edge. I first remember consciously doing this during the Belmont Stakes in June 2004. It was there that I used my penchant for organization and visual stimulation to my advantage. I'd flown across the country to see if Smarty Jones would become the first horse since 1978 to win the Triple Crown.

Years before, it would have been impossible for me to handle a place filled with so many people—more than 120,000 of them, all anxious to catch a glimpse of that red chestnut colt vying for its place in horse-racing history. The lines to everything were long. To make matters worse, cigarette and cigar smoke, smells I loathe, hung heavy in the air. And the noise was deafening. Yet I managed to handle the situation by making games out of every potentially ugly obstacle I encountered. On the line to the portable toilets, I timed the people in front of me, watching to see how long it took them to get in and out of the toilets. I used the same trick at the betting windows and concession lines, which also turned hardship and potential headaches into fun.

On those times when I was forced to wade through a crowd, I turned every step into a game, counting anyone and everyone who resembled Elvis, Alexander Haig, Whoopi Goldberg, and others. That made walking through a sea of people constantly rubbing up against me easier to stomach. In fact, it turned out to be the difference between having a possible meltdown and having a good time. But perhaps my best tactic was something I did long before I arrived at the track, which is a perfect example of an autistic mind at work. I found a map of the racetrack over the Internet and studied it, memorizing the shortest routes from point A to point B, enabling me to get from the racetrack to the exact spot where the horses were being saddled, or from the paddock to the grandstand, in the shortest possible time.

Smarty Jones may have lost that day. But on that particular afternoon, my coping tricks, honed over the course of my lifetime, made me feel like a winner.

TUCSON, ARIZONA
APRIL 2001

Deep down, I truly wanted to give Jerry a white-picket-fence kind of life when we got together for Act Two of our romance. And I almost did. For the first time in years, my head wasn't bothering me. The relative calm and predictability of life in Arizona had somehow quieted the beast between my ears. I was beginning to glimpse the world with amazing clarity, a feat that forced me to realize that all the noise in my head was just that—noise. I realized that I could either focus on the static or accept it for what it was.

And thanks to my on-again-off-again drug regimen of antipsychotics, I finally began to understand how the circuitry inside my head worked—or in my case often didn't. Every time I lost control and the authorities had to be called in, I was ordered to take ever-increasing amounts of medication to correct my neurochemistry. It would work for a while, silencing the crazy thoughts that would erupt from the slightest provocation, then I'd inevitably stop taking them and the madness would begin anew. This pattern repeated itself over and over again. One month I'd be sane, six months later I'd be stark raving mad. This cycle repeated itself so often, over such a compressed period of time, that even someone as thickheaded as me began to understand how all the delusions that had gripped me for so long had been created in the first place. It was like watching dominoes fall—one thing led to the next, over and over and over again. Each crazed fantasy was based on a real event. It was my attempt to create connections, linking one occurrence to the next, trying to find a single common thread that would explain every bit of wrong, every disappointment in my life in one fell swoop. Einstein yearned to create a so-called unified field theory, hoping to resolve the underlying nature of the universe. I wanted to piece together the Asperger's equivalent of it in order to rationalize how all the horrific events of my life were interconnected.

Now that I was beginning to get a better grip on all that internal chatter, I felt myself seized by a single inescapable fact: I was tired of losing everything, tired of the endless cycle of building everything up just so I could tear it down when my neurochemistry went on the fritz. I decided that it was now time to get everything back, to re-create my world.

It was nice, those early days of our second go-round. We were in love all over again, relearning the delicate dance of two very similar yet very different people. We were starting over. And with Peter no longer living with me, Jerry became the main priority of my life.

Back then, Jerry wasn't working. For the first time in years, he was taking some time off while trying to figure out what to do next. After all he'd done for me, my giving him some time to breathe seemed the least I could do. I could tell he desperately wanted to make some changes in his life, to branch off in a new direction. When he finally announced that he wanted to write a book, I thought it sounded like a wonderful idea. It didn't take long for him to line up a publisher, and every day when I'd be at work making sandwiches and pizzas, he'd be typing away on his computer.

Before long, Jerry and I decided to get married again. We'd come this far, so we figured, Why not go all the way? We held our reception at the nearby greyhound racetrack the two of us had been frequenting over the past few months. We'd both come to love the place; it allowed us to utilize a side of our Asperger's that we might never have explored together. It wasn't long before we developed our own unique betting system, one that made full use of our skills. I'd base my criteria solely on how a particular greyhound looked. I watched as the handlers led the dogs onto the track, paying close attention to how each animal walked, the luster of its fur, and how it acted in relation to the other dogs. Jerry based his decision on how each canine looked on paper, crunching his way through whatever statistics he could unearth about any given greyhound. Between my visual prowess of knowing a healthy, energized dog when I saw one and his ability at handicapping, when we could actually agree on a dog to place our money on, we nearly always picked a winner.

In the summer of 2001, I was seized by another one of those ideas I just couldn't shake. I wanted to do more with my life than just make sandwiches and pizza. So I enrolled in cosmetology school and began learning how to put my skills as an artist to work trimming hair. As was typical of me during this peaceful period of my life, I dove headfirst into my studies with a crazed passion. I was ecstatic to have finally discovered a vocation that allowed me to feel like I was making the world a more beautiful place. It was a concept that made me feel better about myself. Yet there was another reason why I so enjoyed helping others change the way they viewed themselves. Years before, during a lull in the chaos and craziness in my life, I'd convinced my parents to let me move back home so I could attend music school at the University of Arizona. Back then, my favorite hobby involved disappearing into our bathroom, locking the door, standing in front of the mirrored doors of the medicine cabinet, and staring intently at the reflection of my face.

I went there to create. The bathroom was my artist's studio. I'd open the door of the cabinet in such a way that I could study the front and side views of my face, trying to reshape it in order to make it look more acceptable, more normal, more like the faces of the people around me. The world had always been an alien place for me. I never fit in. But I'd reached a point in my life where I decided to try. If I was ever going to get anywhere in my life, I told myself that being accepted would be my only hope. If I was going to dissolve into the world, it was crucial that I change how I looked and sounded. So I also practiced speaking, rehearsing lines of dialogue I believed would make me sound more palatable: "You don't say?... That's so wonderful. . . . Maybe sometime the two of us could go get a cup of coffee. . . . I know exactly how you feel." I spent hours working on the way I smiled, trying to tame the muscles around my mouth, trying to tame them to keep them from being so wild and uncontrollably emotive.

My desire to change my face seemed only natural to me. For as long as I could remember, I never felt as though I looked like anyone in my family. Not that I truly ever wanted to. But since I was engaging in all this psychic plastic surgery, I decided to give myself a chin like my father's. Something about the way it jutted out in front of his face like some sturdy bowsprit on a schooner just seemed to command acceptance. And since acceptance was what I craved most, I told myself that if I just concentrated hard enough, I could reshape that part of my face using nothing more than conscious thought. It all seemed fairly simple. On one level, I knew that my chin could be manipulated by the position of my jawbone, which was held in place by various muscles and tendons. That was the easy part. On a deeper level, I knew that my chin, along with the rest of my face, was nothing more than a collection of atoms and molecules, all controlled by electrical forces. In order to manipulate that electrical glue, I would stand in front of the mirror and visualize my face morphing into whatever I willed it to. After awhile, I could feel my cheekbones growing plumper and my eyes becoming more seductive, angel-like in shape.

The more I willed myself into being, the more I censored any thought of my past, the more I enjoyed the new Mary. Yet every so often I'd feel a slight twinge of doubt ripple through my body, reminding me that I couldn't run forever, that one day my carefully constructed façade would crumble. Exactly who the real Mary was, I pretended not to care. Why should I? I was having too much fun with the new and improved version.

Nine months after starting, I graduated from beauty college, then passed my state licensing test and hit the streets looking for work. I felt positively high, like there was nothing I couldn't accomplish if I put my mind to it. Originally, I considered taking a job at a trendy salon in Tucson. But I soon realized I didn't fit in there— my tastes were a bit more grounded than the latest coifs coming out of Paris, New York, and Los Angeles. So I went to work at a simple barbershop frequented by vets from World War II, Korea, and Vietnam. They were a tough, grizzled lot, many of whom still carried pieces of shrapnel in their bodies. None of them gave a rat's ass about the latest style of haircut I'd spent months learning at school. All they wanted were the kinds of cuts that had been in existence for decades—crew cuts, flattops, fade cuts. From the moment I stepped into that dusty, old barbershop, I felt at home with these old warriors. We were all survivors.

I liked it there. I'd cut their hair and we'd swap stories about the battles we'd both fought. Over time, however, I noticed that it was becoming increasingly difficult to make accurate cuts with my scissors and electric trimmers. The more I tried to relax, the more my body would seize up. The doctors suspected that my medications were the cause. So I stopped taking them, reasoning that since I finally seemed to be in control of my life for the first time in years, what could it hurt? Something close to happiness was welling up inside of me. I was achieving my goals and in love again. If nothing was wrong with me, why on earth did I need medication?

It only took a few months before I found out.

Off and on for the next few years, I drifted in and out of a handful of mental institutions. I'd bottom out, then just as I hit rock bottom my heavily medicated brain would snap back like a rubber band. Eventually, I began to understand the role Lars played in my delusions, about how the aircraft flying over our house uncaged all those awful memories of being held captive by him in the desert.

On the day I told Jerry of my breakthrough, the muscles around his eyes twitched and something about the shape of his mouth led me to believe that a lightbulb had flashed on inside his head. So I ran into my bedroom and grabbed a tattered copy of the Diagnostics Statistics Manual IV I'd been poring over for the past few weeks. I opened it to the pages that described my condition—posttraumatic stress disorder—and handed it to Jerry. He read it over and over again. Afterward, he sat down on the sofa and ran his fingers through his dirty hair.

"Yeah," he mumbled slowly, as it all sank into his brain. "This really sounds like you, Mary." He didn't move for a long time. He just stared down at the pages, then whispered, "I'm . . . I'm sorry."

At first, I thought he was just trying to be polite. "Yeah, it really sucks being crazy," I replied.

"No . . . no," he said, looking up into my eyes. "I'm sorry for what I did, for all the yelling. You've had it rough in this life, Mary. Far, far rougher than me." Jerry paused for a moment and I could see that he had tears in his eyes. "Up until now, I . . . I just never realized how all these pieces from your life—your family, Lars, the Children of God—fit together to cause you so much pain. If I could take it all back, I would. But I can't. I can only promise that I'll never yell around you again."

And he never did. After that day, Jerry never raised his voice around me. I don't know how he did it. Autistic tantrums aren't something you can just turn off like you would a water faucet. When one explodes inside you, all you can do is hold on, let it rip, and pray that whoever is within earshot is either understanding or deaf.

One morning not long after that, Jerry announced, "You know, there really is a movie."

"What?" I stammered, not quite sure what I was hearing.

"A movie," he said. "There really is a movie. Spielberg really did buy the rights to our movie."

I stood there staring at him, not quite sure what to say. Months before, I'd forced myself to ignore any thoughts or memories I had of my dealings with Hollywood. For him to tell me suddenly that there really was a movie after all, that all the psychologists, therapists, and social workers who tried to convince me that I was delusional for daring to think such a thing were wrong, seemed so . . . so like a strange joke, the kind with no punch line.

Sort of like my life.

CHAPTER ELEVEN

If I had to think back to the perfect Jerry-Mary moment, the first one that comes to mind involves a little game the two of us began playing shortly after moving out to our house in the desert. It was a spontaneous sort of thing. And since spontaneity is a concept that neither of our brains is particularly good at grasping, this particular game of ours has always smacked of pure magic.

The moment always began the same way: Mary would be sitting on the sofa with our cockatiel Shayna perched on her shoulder and I'd walk into the room. The moment Shayna spotted me, she'd flap her wings a few times, flutter across the room, and land on my head. Having a bird on my head always made me feel as though I were wearing a crown of feathers. Which is why I'd always just stand there, looking at Mary, then shout, "I am the bird god!"

No matter how hard she tried to fight it, Mary would inevitably throw back her head and roar with laughter.

"No, you're not!" she'd scream.

Almost on cue, I'd feel Shayna's tiny talons pinch into my scalp;

then she'd launch herself airborne and traverse the space between the two of us, always landing back on Mary's shoulder.

"Now I'm the bird god!" Mary would shriek. "And don't you forget it!"

We could play this game for a half hour or so, until Shayna would get bored with us and fly off to join the other birds sunning themselves in a back bedroom.

Something clicked inside me during the summer of 2003. I've never quite understood why it happened when it did. Maybe it was the first time I really tried to listen to what was lurking behind Mary's crazy words, instead of just doing my best to tolerate them. It happened late one afternoon as Mary began her usual rant about how the helicopters that sometimes flew over our house were causing her head to fill with all those awful memories of her days spent as Lars's prisoner out in the Arizona desert near some army base. Somewhere in the middle of her pained rant, which I knew by heart, she mentioned something called PTSD—short for posttraumatic stress disorder. Of course, I'd heard of this condition before. A couple of men in AGUA claimed to suffer from it due to the traumas they'd endured while being bullied in school. They used to tell me how certain things, such as the sound of someone shouting, could trigger memories of their terrible childhood torture sessions.

A few hours after my conversation with Mary, I drove to a nearby library and started reading up on PTSD. The more I learned, the more I had to admit that it certainly sounded like Mary, especially the part about how a simple stimulus can cause people with this disorder to relive their traumas and how it can ultimately warp their perception of reality. That next morning when Mary finally dragged herself out of bed, she told me that when I yelled at her, it reminded her of how Lars used to treat her.

That was all I needed to hear.

I never yelled at Mary again after that. And I apologized for all the pain my shouting had caused her. Up until that moment, I'd always viewed yelling as manly tradition in the Newport family. My father was a major-league yeller. I regarded it as nothing more than an emotional release. But once Mary calmly made me understand how my thunderous voice affected her, I put a sock in it. As corny as it sounds, I could feel her pain and all I wanted to do was make it stop. It's a lot like what happened twenty years ago, when I finally decided to quit smoking. After going through a particularly disgusting spell of spitting gunk out from my lungs, I said to myself: To hell with this, I'm not smoking anymore. And that was all it took.

I can be a thickheaded guy. But once I finally understand that something might be harmful to myself or others, I have no choice but to change my behavior. To do otherwise wouldn't be logical. And it certainly wouldn't be autistic.

Despite the good times and my occasional epiphanies, our daily life together still sometimes resembled a roller-coaster ride at Six Flags. Which was why I began to relish the respite brought on by my out-of-town speaking gigs. And it was in those hotel ballrooms and convention halls that I began to notice another type of shift occurring deep inside me. This time it involved my sense of identity. Suddenly, instead of feeling myself drawn to people with Asperger's, I started spending more time thinking about what it must feel like to be the parent of an Aspie. (On more than a few occasions, after observing how the parents behaved at these seminars, it was sometimes difficult to tell them apart from their children.) Before long, I'd begun using my talks as a way to help these mothers and fathers begin to see that life is for living, tasting, touching, and biting into. I spoke repeatedly about the importance of finding situations and places where their kids could share their interests, no matter how simple or outrageously complex, with others.

"Forget about team sports like basketball," I'd explain. "Get your kids involved in things like Cub Scouts, science or math clubs, musical organizations. Those are the places where I met most of my friends."

Of course, I wasn't the guy who dreamed up that advice. My father did. That was his philosophy. He used it on me when he saw what a hard time I was having with life. The more I pondered my father's memory, the more I began to appreciate his tough-love approach to making me a man. And it made me wonder: how many others who had tried to reach out to me had I ignored or rebuffed? Some days, it hurt to think about how I'd squandered the time I'd had with him. He'd tried his best to get close to me, but I'd pushed him away. He deserved better than that. Sure, he got frustrated with me at times, terribly so. But without a doubt he's one of the main reasons why I've managed to make anything out of my life. His motto was: Always do the right thing, but never expect to get recognition for doing it.

Not long ago, I put a twist on that motto. In a way, I suppose you could say it's my motto now. It goes like this: If you want to be a hero on earth, don't expect any credit in the hereafter. This is what I've tried to do over the last part of my life—tried my best to help my peers. Yet despite my best intentions, there's a bit of guilt attached to being the guy who helped popularize the concept of autistic-to-autistic marriage. The union between Mary and me has apparently even led some people within our community to believe that the best possible way to solve the troubling problem of isolation among autistic adults simply is to marry us all off to one another. In recent years, the idea has been bandied about in various Internet chat groups and discussed at conferences. In my opinion this suggestion, no matter how well intended, is a laughable, knee-jerk reaction to a dilemma that many non-Aspies wish would just go away.

The flaws with this solution are far too numerous to list. And the statistical issue of the reported four-to-one male-to-female ratio is hardly the biggest hurdle. (After all, why not legalize reverse polygamy and allow each autistic female to have four husbands!)

Seriously, the main barrier is this: even if there were a one-to-one male-to-female ratio, most men and women with autism are too similarly challenged to do each other much good as partners.

Friends, absolutely.

But marriage? Rarely.

Why? I can only offer a few observations I gleaned from my years running AGUA, which gave me a priceless in-the-trenches look at the collective differences between autistic men and women. For starters, female AGUA members normally possess much more social experience than their male counterparts. Just ask those women who *risked* attending an AGUA meeting and had the pleasure of being stampeded by a roomful of clueless autistic guys. Nearly every female in AGUA had a boyfriend or two in her past by the time she found her way to our group. Most had been married, and more than half had children. Two were actually grandmothers.

The male side of the picture is just the opposite—in the extreme. Most AGUA men, even those in their thirties or older, have never embarked upon a single date in their lives. And if they have somehow managed to go out with a woman on occasion, it's been years since such an occurrence has repeated itself. Girlfriends? Maybe 10 percent have had one. Marriage? So far, two guys out of eighty members have tied the knot—although one of them was apparently suckered into an arranged marriage by a South American mail-order bride scheme. The woman hit the road the moment her U.S. citizenship came through.

"And she even kept the ring," moaned her abandoned husband at an AGUA meeting shortly after she skipped out on him.

So what's really behind this depressing trend? My guess, from what I've heard, is that the inherent social naïveté of autistic women often allows them to get sucked into relationships. Rarely are these liaisons good ones. Compounding the problem is that the low self-image they share with their male peers keeps them in these unhealthy relationships and marriages for far too long.

The bottom line is clear: autistic women manage to get a taste of social interaction that males don't. This puts them light-years ahead of their male counterparts.

Other gender-related autistic traits factor into the equation a bit differently. For instance, a passive woman is attractive to many men, yet a passive male is a turnoff to most women. Hundreds of thousands of years may have elapsed since our species lived in caves and killed food with spears, but our collective view of how men and women are supposed to behave has changed little. Whether we want to admit it or not, men are still viewed as the designated hunters and, as ridiculous as it sounds, women play the role of the prize.

I've never put much faith in the so-called four-to-one ratio touted by many experts. I've always felt that autism is seen more in men because basic autistic traits tend to run counter to the accepted way our culture believes men are supposed to behave. In other words, autism is just easier to detect in males. The ratio—whatever it really is—isn't the point. The real issue is that our community is filled with a group of men who are *expected* to be leading the dance. Yet they are so scared of attempting even a single step that the more experienced women in our midst aren't interested in putting up with their glaring shortcomings. Not surprisingly, when an Aspie woman goes searching for male company, she's going to look for someone who is focused, sincere, tactilely patient, and orderly. Sure, maybe he'll have some oddities that parallel autism, but at least he'll be able to perform the social requirements expected of him, a feat that baffles and scares so many of my male peers. These include being able to initiate action (such as a conversation or, God forbid, a date), knowing how to follow up afterward, being attentive, and not being freaked out by physical intimacy.

If I had to write out the dialogue that one might typically hear at the tail end of a date between an autistic male and a female, here's how it would go:

She: (*Thinking to herself: Is he going to try to touch me? Does he know how and when?*) So ... ?

He: Uhhhh ... So, what do you want to do now?

She: You don't really seem to know what you want to do. So maybe I should be going home.

He: (*With a sigh of relief*) Okay. See you later.

Or, how about the dialogue between an autistic man telephoning a woman to ask for date:

He: Hello, is Peggy there?

She: Speaking.

He: Uh, uh, uh . . . You wouldn't want to see *Men in Black* with me, would you?

She: I guess not.

He: Yeah, that's what I thought. I'll talk to you later. Goodbye.

When I shared those scenarios during a recent conference, some people wrote me off as an insensitive creep. And that frustrated me. They were missing the point I was hoping to make. Which was this: If we're ever going to change the current sad state of things, we need to face the truth. And that truth is grim, if not worse. Most autistic guys don't even get the chance to fail. They're too petrified to even try. Why? It's not due to a lack of interest in members of the opposite sex. The reason is pure, utter cluelessness—either too much or not enough. Which is why so many of our guys get in trouble for staring and other "stalking"-type behavior that gets them fired from jobs, arrested, or both.

I'll never forget New Year's Eve in 1995 when Mary and I organized an AGUA party attended mostly by men. The highlight of the evening was when her youngest son, Peter, then nineteen, stopped by while en route to another party with two women

friends. The moment those two young women entered our apartment, you could feel the one-sided sexual tension ricocheting off
the walls. Every guy in the room just stood there, staring at these
two females. After a few tense minutes, the men began pacing
about like caged, nervous animals. Then, almost as if driven by
some silent signal, they closed ranks and charged, circling their
prey en masse.

Peter and his two friends fled the party not long after that.

The next day, Mary bumped into the girls and asked them what
they thought of the AGUA men. They looked at each other and
smiled, then rolled their eyes. "No foreplay!" they shouted.

When you get right down to it, it doesn't matter if you're an early
bloomer, a normal bloomer, or a late bloomer. What's important
is that you don't pass through this life without ever blooming.
Which brings me to my theory: I have a hunch that Mary asked me
out on that first date in 1994 because she realized that I was a man
in the midst of blossoming, the kind of guy who called the shots
in his life. She certainly didn't ask me out because she thought I
had a lot of money. After all, I was a deliveryman who didn't even
own a car. Was it my appearance? I seriously doubt that. Half the
time, my hopelessly wrinkled clothes were covered with smears of
ketchup and other stains. My hunch is that what attracted Mary
to me was that she could sense that I—for better or worse—was
trying to make it through life on my own, setting my own course
and not making any excuses when I occasionally crashed and
burned. And that's the ultimate sexual turn-on, something I believe means more to a woman than possibly anything else.

I'm convinced that anyone can learn to become a shot caller
in their own life if they just keep playing the game long enough.
It's a skill that just takes time and plenty of patience. Which is
one of the reasons why I keep trying to do my part to help those
generations of Aspies who are just entering the game (along with

their caregivers), to give them an honest assessment of the terrain that lies before them. And my advice is this: whether you're an autistic man or woman, you're going to be a social late bloomer. So don't sweat it. Like it or not, most of us lack the superficial skills that make people popular in high school or even college. Yet as time goes by, our true qualities—honesty, reliability, sincerity, and focus—become more attractive. That goes a long way in explaining why it took me forty-six years before my first marriage, even with an above-average IQ, a mainstream education, and a hefty amount of social experience that was much more "normal" than that of my peers.

This much is true: we will never cure the isolation of autism by marrying off all our autistic men and women. If they get married at all, and if it is to be a good marriage, it will only happen after they learn to love and accept themselves first. Then, and only then, does it make sense to try to seek a complementary, compatible partner. Just don't expect them to be autistic—although they might possess a few autistic traits.

The way I see it, life is stuffed full of surprises. The moment you drop your guard, the road you're traveling down makes one of those hairpin turns that you never quite see coming. Our impulsive decision to move to a five-acre spread out in the desert was like that. It came out of the blue and we never regretted it for an instant. For the first time in our lives, we both realized what a godsend quiet could be. The calm did wonders for Mary's head and my nerves. Our relationship wasn't perfect, but it was far better than it ever had been.

I was giving Mary more space now, which felt nice for both of us. I'd finally begun to understand that I didn't need to be around somebody all the time in order to enjoy their companionship. That wasn't the case during our first marriage. Back then, I went out of my way to smother Mary with my attention. After all, I'd finally found my soul mate. The last thing I wanted to do was let her slip through my fingers because of inattentiveness. (I did the same thing with houseplants on those rare occasions I found myself in possession of one—I'd love it to death with constant, daily watering.)

I can still remember the day Mary told me she'd joined the church choir near our apartment in Santa Monica. I felt so uneasy about it that the next afternoon when I got off work, despite not having a lick of interest in singing, I joined the choir, too. Why not? I thought. Why shouldn't we share every single aspect of our lives with each other? For an autistic person in love for the first time in his life, that sort of thinking made perfect sense.

On another occasion, I decided to telephone Mary from my desk at UCLA . . . a few times, just to "check up" on her. Since I knew she never left the apartment, I couldn't understand why she wouldn't answer the phone. So during my lunch break I sped over to our apartment to make sure she was all right, to convince myself that she hadn't packed up her belongings and fled.

"Why didn't you answer the phone?" I screamed when I ran into the apartment and found her staring out the window, hypnotized by the swaying lilac-blue branches of a jacaranda tree in the courtyard. After snapping out of her trance, she looked at me with a dazed, wide-eyed look that soon turned to annoyance.

"I just unplugged the phone, Jerry," she moaned. "You gotta back off. I can't breathe when you do this."

These days, I don't need to be around Mary as much as I did. All I know is that it's finally just enough to know she's there, somewhere in our home, loving our animals in the same crazy way I do, and killing time with the same effortless skill that I possess—a feat that involves not doing anything for hours on end and not feeling a scrap of guilt about it. One thing's certain: Mary finally taught me to love and appreciate my inner couch potato. The hours we spend sitting around, watching TV, joking about the ridiculous stupidity and implausibility of whatever program we happen to be viewing while our birds and iguanas run through the house, are priceless.

One of the things we both get a kick out of is ribbing each other about our much-hyped movie. Not too long ago, it became something of a silent running joke between the two of us. We'd resigned ourselves to the fact that it was probably never going to see the light of day. Then one morning the telephone rang in our kitchen. I picked it up and heard an officious-sounding voice announce: "I have producer Robert Lawrence on the line. Hold please."

"Who is it?" Mary asked.

"It's Hollywood," I informed her. "They've tracked us down again."

She rolled her eyes and laughed. "Hang up," she begged.

I shook my head. Over the course of the next few minutes, Robert informed me that our script had finally gotten the green light. Filming would begin in a few months. Before hanging up, he added, "I've got someone here who wants to talk to you. He's going to play you in the movie."

"Hi," a voice said. "I'm Josh. It's great to speak with you."

"Josh who?" I asked.

"Josh . . . Hartnett," he insisted. "I'm really excited about this project."

We spoke for a few minutes, exchanged phone numbers, then I put the phone down.

"Who was that?" Mary inquired.

"Josh Hartnett," I told her. "He's going to play me in the movie."

"That's nice, Jerry," she said. "We need more bird seed."

Whatever happens to the two of us, I couldn't have asked for a better teacher than Mary. She's forced me to grow in ways I never dreamed possible, convinced me to stop imagining that the world revolves around me. Finally becoming part of a real relationship, one where

I got to care for someone and am cared for by the other, has worked some kind of strange magic over me. It has helped forge me into a better person. Sure, there are plenty of times when I overreacted, plenty of opportunities where I should have behaved differently. But Mary was the first woman who made me feel like I wasn't stepping on eggshells when I was around her, like I didn't have to make myself into another person in order for someone to like me.

Mary has allowed me to become more comfortable with being Jerry Newport. Who could ask for a better gift than that? Sure, there's a part of me that will forever remain an awkward sixteen-year-old, starved for attention, desperate for acceptance, hungry for love. But little by little, day by day, he has begun to grow up. Which reminds me of the one lesson I've learned from this crazy life of mine: happily ever after doesn't exist for anyone, especially for those of us with Asperger's. We were born in an unusual way, with unusual traits. Like it or not, we're never going to fit into the so-called normal world. (Sometimes I wonder why anyone would want to.)

You can deny this fact of life all you want. You can pretend it doesn't hold true for you or your child. But sooner or later, you'll have to accept it. And, the funny thing is, once you do that, something magical happens deep inside you. You start to accept who it is you really are. And you begin to forge a friendship with the most special, wonderful person you can ever meet—yourself.

BENSON, ARIZONA
MAY 2003

The universe works in strange ways: just when you think the jig is up, you get a second chance. One sweltering afternoon in May 2003, a stranger appeared on our front doorstep and, instead of slapping him—like I did years earlier when a lawyer arrived to deliver a check from DreamWorks—I invited him inside. I love listening to salesmen, following the arc of their pitch as they try to sweep you up with their words and carry you away. He'd come to offer us cash for our house, but we somehow ended up swapping houses with him instead.

Moving out to the desert was probably one of the most logical, sensible things I've ever done. From the moment we arrived, the quiet and calm wrapped itself around us like a blanket. Often the only sound comes from the wind blowing across the sand and rock. Sometimes Jerry drives past and toots the horn of his cab, which he began driving not long after we moved here. It's nearly impossible to get your brain overstimulated in a place like this.

Soon after we moved in, I took a job at a salon in a nearby military town. It didn't go well. The owner wanted me to cut hair the way an assembly-line worker attaches widget A to widget B. All he cared about was efficiency and speed—*chop, chop, chop. Next customer.* But I always viewed myself as an artist, someone who needed time to create. Unfortunately, when he saw how slow I was, he grew angry and frustrated with me, which soon caused me to shake and grow terribly nervous. After only two weeks on the job, he fired me.

"It's not enough to know what sets me off," I told Jerry when I arrived home after getting sacked. "I have to know what to avoid."

Jerry smiled and patted me on the back. He didn't say a word. He didn't have to.

Lately, I don't feel the need to paint that much anymore. I'm sure I'll get the hankering back someday. Perhaps that otherworldly muse who has always guided my hand when I paint is allowing me to rest up before my next explosion of creativity. Mostly, I just enjoy sitting in the front room of our house while the sun comes streaming in through the windows. I puff on my Marlboro and will myself to dissolve, to fade into the background in order to better observe our animals entertaining themselves.

It's peculiar, I think, that this room is one of the only places where I've ever felt safe enough to want to dissolve. At the same time, it's also one of the few places I've never wanted to leave. I love it here, especially the quiet. After all these years, my sensitive ears have grown tired of noise. What I enjoy most is the sound that the tiny feet of our animals make as they tear through the house—the cockatiel chasing the dog, who chases the cat, who chases the iguana, who chases the cockatiel.

In the afternoons, I can stare out the windows for hours at the massive, tired mountains jutting up from the high desert that surrounds us. A menagerie of animals parades through our brush-strewn property—quail, javelina, deer, and wild rabbits. One of those rabbits, with fur the color of an old pair of beat-up cowboy boots I used to own, loves to tease our dog, Cujoy. Deep inside his little rabbit brain, he seems to know that Cujoy is tied up to a leash, so he runs as close as he can to him, then leaps high into the air at the last possible moment.

Some days I can just make out the soft rumble of railcars miles away from our house. Jerry loves to drive out there, to the railroad crossing out near the Circle K convenience store, and count the train cars filled with Chinese-labeled freight as they roll past. Once he comes up with the number, he begins running it through his head and it makes me smile to think of him out there, parked on the side of the road, weaving order and meaning out of something as arbitrary as how many railcars he happened to count rolling past him.

Not long ago, I began asking myself where all *this* was heading. Not my life. I've long ago stopped trying to plot the course that was going to take. What I really wonder about is what's going to become of people like Jerry and me. Over the past few years, I've caught rumblings (in books, on the Internet, and within our community) that we autistics are prototypes for a new kind of human—we're the latest branch on the evolutionary tree, neurologically unlike the majority of humanity. Which makes sense to me. In fact, the more I think about it, the prouder I feel to be standing with my boots firmly planted at the fork in the road of evolution. Because if this planet of ours—along with our species—has any chance of surviving, it's time we try something new, genetically. A few tweaks of the DNA could probably do all of us a world of good. It certainly couldn't hurt, since we've managed to make such a mess of things over the past few thousand years.

I call this new human, for whom Jerry and I serve as the proud flag bearers, *homo cognitas*. And I imagine him/her to possess two somewhat diametrically opposed qualities: an unquenchable desire to organize and identify the underlying structure of the universe coupled with copious amounts of empathy. The way I see it, *homo cognitas* will be a cross between Mr. Spock and Gandhi. Don't laugh. I'm convinced that the human brain, every aberrational twist and turn it has taken over the past few million or so years, is all part of a long-term experiment that we're all part of, that essentially started with the Big Bang. With every child born comes the chance that some random permutation inside their brain—whether it be autism or something else—will provide the key to unlock the next door we're supposed to pass through. We're creeping forward, all of us, axon by axon, dendrite by dendrite, to a future not even I can imagine. But—when all is quiet and my mind is right—I can sometimes catch glimpses of it.

That is, of course, until Jerry comes stomping into the house and shouting: "Fifty-three!"

To which I reply: "Okay, fifty-three what?"

"The number painted on the side of all those railcars," Jerry says. "You ever noticed how all the railcars that come roaring through here have the number fifty-three painted on them? Well, I finally figured out what it all means."

Jerry looks at me, cracks that adorable goofy smile of his, and I love him more in that moment than I ever knew possible. And I feel that mysterious glue that holds us together welling up inside me. It tickles and I think to myself: I love the way love feels.

But by this point, Jerry is off, traipsing through his land of numbers. "Those cars are fifty-three feet long," he gushes. "That's what the number fifty-three is all about. That works out to about one hundred cars per mile. So, if it takes four locomotives to pull it, that means there would be ninety-six train cars. You know what I love about the number ninety-six? It's what you get when you take two to the fifth power, then multiply that by three. . . . And fifty-three is a great number if you're into Corvettes—1953 was the year they introduced them."

"You don't say," I reply, faking a yawn.

Jerry grins, and, out of absolutely nowhere, shouts: "Let's drive to Tombstone!"

"Tombstone?" I ask.

"Yeah," he says. "We've been talking about doing it for the past couple of weeks. Let's get in the car and go. I'm all ready."

By saying he's all ready, Jerry actually means he's got every single iota of the trip all plotted out on a map, mile by mile, signpost by signpost. By doing that, he knows he'll never have to ask me for directions, a lapse in judgment that always ended up sending Jerry into a rage whenever we'd go on road trips during our first marriage. He doesn't yell at me anymore and even lets me place my hand on his shoulder as the two of us listen to one of Bach's fugues trickling out of the radio. It's a beautiful ride down to Tombstone, through the tattered outskirts of Benson, past the local animal hospital—where we just spent nearly all our savings paying for our iguana to undergo stomach surgery—and into the town of St. David, which spreads out before us like a quilt of wet, green grass.

By the time we hit Tombstone, the first thing we want to see is the Boot Hill Cemetery. But we decide to exhibit a bit of restraint and park on the other end of town, so we can walk to Main Street and save the dead people for last.

"I need a whiskey, Jerry," I announce after hopping out of the car. So we walk into Big Nose Kate's Saloon and I order a shot of bourbon, then toss it back. It burns a trail all the way down into my gut. "Gimme one more," I tell the barkeep and watch as something magical happens to Jerry's face. It softens and all at once I know he's okay with my playing out my cowgirl fantasy.

"I'm gonna go get a sandwich," he laughs. "Meet you in the graveyard in an hour."

"Make it two hours," I tell him, gazing out at the colorful crowd seated around me, sucking down drinks. "I want to hang out with these locals for a bit."

Jerry wanders out of the saloon, out into bright, dusty daylight, and I experience that feeling again, flopping around inside my chest like a drunken squid—love. My version of it.

A few more shots of bourbon and an order of pork rinds later, I wander down Main Street and spot Jerry gazing at a group of street musicians grinning and picking on their banjos. I take his large hand in mine and squeeze it. We stand there and listen to a screeching ballad about love gone terribly wrong. As the music plays, I tap my foot against the wooden boardwalk and watch a cloud of dust drift over the toe of my boot. When it's all over, we continue walking down Main Street, all the way to the Boot Hill Cemetery, and wander among the rock-strewn plots containing the brittle bones of people who were long ago killed in stagecoach robberies, mine-shaft explosions, arguments while playing cards, even the occasional tomahawk. Something about all this tragedy makes me jealous—death was so much more exciting and dramatic back then.

Over the next half hour, we read our way through that cemetery, moving from one weathered wooden marker to the next, pausing to absorb the sad, peculiar epitaphs: Here Lies Lester Moore / Four Slugs from a 44 / No Les / No More. Here Lies George Johnson / Hanged by Mistake 1882 / He Was Right / We Was Wrong / But We Strung Him Up / And Now He's Gone. Johnny Blair / Died of Smallpox / Cowboy Threw Rope Over Feet and Dragged Him to His Grave.

Jerry didn't say much for most of the drive back to our house in Benson. He was thinking about something. I could tell by the way he squinted, how the skin around his eyes rippled and creased into a maze of soft furrows.

"I've got it," he says, finally breaking the silence.

"Got what, Jerry?" I ask.

"An epitaph," he laughs. "I know how I want my epitaph to read."

"How's that?" I reply.

Jerry turns, looks straight into my eyes for a few moments. He doesn't even blink. And, for some reason, it never occurs to me to be nervous, despite the fact that he's the one driving. "Living was a good idea," he says. "I hope to do it again."

When Jerry and I first met, I'd spent most of my life searching for the kind of love that existed only in greeting cards. I don't know if that was due to the artist—or the autistic—in me. But these days I'm much more practical. Maybe it takes losing everything to finally transform the way you see the world. Or maybe some of Jerry is just rubbing off on me. All I know is that my raison d'être these days is to have a friend with whom I can negotiate my life, someone to walk with for what's left of my journey here.

When I compare what we have now with what we had before, I see that most of what got lost or screwed up the first time around has been fixed. Back then, Jerry didn't pick up on my nonverbal signals. And so much of what I do when I'm stressed is nonverbal. I turn off all the lights, pull down the shades, and retreat deep inside of myself. And when I did that, Jerry always wanted to follow me inside. He'd pound on the door and when I didn't answer, he'd kick it in. Which is the last thing a woman like me needs. He doesn't do that anymore.

These days, Jerry watches as best he can for any sort of signal from me, any type of visual cue that I'm in distress, then he backs off. I do the same thing with him. It's rarely easy, but when I feel my blood pressure rising, I take a few breaths before letting loose with my tongue or before allowing myself to float away. More often than not, that's all it takes to cool myself down, to get a sense of perspective that used to be missing when the moment heated up. Giving someone an extra second or two to think or relax may not sound like a big deal, but for people like us it's a critical extra couple of seconds, the difference between feeling like you're sleeping with the enemy and sleeping with a friend.

Another thing I've come to realize is that, despite my eccentric, artsy outer shell, I'm more of a one-track person than Jerry. That's definitely saying something because Jerry is a textbook example of a monorail. I just keep it a bit more hidden than he does. And unlike him, I don't fly into a rage when my train of thought gets derailed. I shut down. Looking back on our first marriage, I'm sure that even he could detect the distress in my eyes and in the way I held my body. Yet he rarely got it—at least not when it really mattered. All that has changed now. Being alone with our problems for those years when we'd broken up finally forced us to look at ourselves in a way we never had before. We're learning from each other, Jerry and I.

We both have an equal commitment not to offend each other. We both understand that we can't assume the other person is going to automatically accept everything we do or say. That means we have to show each other more consideration than we did in the past. We can't tromp around on each other's hearts and feelings the way we used to. Having Asperger's doesn't give anyone the right to act like the proverbial bull in the china shop. Whether we like it or not, there are certain things that will never get resolved between us and we've come to accept that. Which is the real mystery of love: being okay with that which makes your other half unique and different from you.

On any given morning at our house, those *differences* often come crashing down upon our heads with the force of a hurled brick. For example, Jerry is an early riser; I, on the other hand, have always enjoyed sleeping until the crack of noon whenever the opportunity presents itself. Jerry is also one of those people whose brain wakes up the moment his body does. He's fully cranked and humming the moment he opens his eyes. The first thing Jerry does each morning is just lie there and watch me sleep. He focuses on me so intently that I can almost feel the pressure of his eyes burning a hole in my body. This morning ritual of his used to creep me out when we first met. I'd never experienced such a thing before. Most people couldn't stand looking at me when I was awake, when I was doing everything I could to pretend I was normal. It never occurred to me that anyone would want to look when I wasn't even awake.

"Look at her, she even sleeps like one of those autistics!" I imagined them sneering.

But not Jerry. For as long as I could remember, I went to sleep knowing that for the next few hours all I had to do was keep my eyes shut and the world, which had never wanted anything to do with me, would thankfully disappear. Yet, to fall sleep each night and know that before I awoke, somebody would gaze upon my still body and feel thankful to be in my presence . . . well, it definitely took some getting used to.

After gazing at me snoring the morning away, Jerry would usually hop in the shower and I'd pull the pillow over my head to block out the noise the water made pounding against the tub. Next, he'd clang around the kitchen, making breakfast and listening to the news on TV. That was his way of rousing me in the morning, but it never worked. So he'd wander into our bedroom and say something like: "Mary, it's almost noon. We were going to catch the 12:15 matinee in town. You better get up."

I'd reply by moaning and pulling the pillow down tighter around my head.

"Mary," Jerry would say. "I've fed the birds and the lizards, but we need rabbit food. Didn't you just get rabbit food the other day?... Or did you tell *me* to get rabbit food?" By this point, I'd usually be forced to insert my fingers into my ears in order to drown out Jerry's voice.

But here's the rub: during our first marriage, Jerry's annoying morning-person traits would have easily pushed me over the edge. Now, on those occasions when he's all perky and chatty and I'm still trying to catch some shut-eye, I take a deep breath and remind myself: That's just my Jerry.

And then I fall back asleep.

Another maddening *tendency* of my husband's that used to drive me nuts is his insatiable need to sit on our sofa and scribble out intricate lists, schedules, and outlines of all the various projects he wants to undertake. His list-making condition is so acute that the other day I caught him making a list of all his other lists.

"It just helps me keep track of things in my head." He laughed, looking almost embarrassed to be caught in the act. Although it doesn't bother me anymore, that trait once annoyed me so horribly I'd want to pull out my hair. In the time I've known him, Jerry could fill a library with all of his lists. Yet I couldn't make one if my life depended on it. I wouldn't know where to start. I'm more of a drifter. I float from one activity to the next like a cloud. My concept of time is much less solid than Jerry's. For me, the world feels so airy and vaporous that it's no wonder I'm prone to floating away when things turn ugly. Jerry's infernal to-do lists seem almost like an anchor, and that's the last thing I want to be carrying around.

Something else I've come to understand about my husband is that the advice he's so stuffed full of stems from his real desire to help people lead the kind of life he only recently learned how to experience. It's no wonder he's been asked to travel the world to dispense some of what he's learned in life to people in our community. I was thinking about him the other day while I was spacing out, looking at a piece of tumbleweed blowing past our front yard. It hit me, if I had any advice to pass on to others, it would be this: Being in a relationship with another autistic person can be a mixed blessing, one that provides you with the most wonderful gifts imaginable, along with the most dizzying challenges. To make it work, you not only have to share those gifts with each other, you also have to be committed to tackling whatever problems arise.

One big difference between our second marriage and our first is that Jerry and I share our respective savant skills with each other instead of guarding them so jealously. I teach Jerry new things about my art, how certain mixtures of colors, images, or sounds create different impressions on people. He teaches me about numbers, allowing me glimpses of how the world is really just one massive combination of quantities.

I don't get out all that much anymore. I certainly don't travel the way Jerry does. But I suspect that there are many more couples out there like Jerry and me. If I ever got to give one of those talks like he does, here's what I'd tell those people out there like Jerry and me, who are trying to make their relationships work: Get a shoe box, decorate it up, and turn it into a treasure chest. Next, write down all the things that you and your mate love to do together on scraps of paper and place those scraps inside your treasure chest. Then, find a trash can, write down all your negative traits—not necessarily what you've been told not to like, but what it is that doesn't make you feel good about yourself. Toss all those scraps into the wastebasket. The last thing you need to do is ask yourself this simple question: What would I rather do—dig through a treasure chest or rummage through a trash can?

So much has changed between Jerry and me over these past few years. The atmosphere between us is no longer so unbearably dense. It's easier to drag the air into my lungs. It's more nourishing. Like most of the things that give meaning to that time we're given between birth and death, these changes have mostly been subtle—at least when you try to picture them with a *normal* mind. In our first marriage, Jerry eventually became so sensitive to touch that hugging him was like trying to wrap my arms around a cactus. Which is why I loved having all those cactuses growing around my house in Tucson after we split up. They reminded me of Jerry and why I'd left him. Yet, over time, the incredible beauty of those hearty plants—which can withstand so much and ask for so little—reminded me of what I loved about him. They were not only survivors, but they provided sustenance for me at a time when I had very little else.

Jerry is just like that. As long as he's a part of my life, I know that even at my lowest point, even when I have nowhere else to turn, he'll be there for me, waiting to give me the nourishment I need to continue on. And after he moved out here to be with me, to start over, it didn't take long before I noticed that removing Los Angeles from his system transformed Jerry back into my lovable teddy bear.

Here's something else I realized not so long ago about us. Back when we first met, the two of us were filled with so much anger over our lives that it tore us apart. Unresolved anger lay at the root of everything we did, every word we spoke. It festered inside us, lurking like a thief in an alley, waiting to spoil anything good that might happen. The ironic thing is, my anger really had nothing to do with Jerry and his had nothing to do with me. It was a residue from our pasts, built up from lifetimes of frustration. With counseling at an early stage in our relationship, the kind of couples' therapy that could have allowed each of us to understand and express this emotion that was eating us up, we might have had a chance.

Not long before we decided to get remarried, Jerry and I made the decision to finally, consciously attempt to excise all that wrath from our lives. We'd come to understand that the only way our union would work was if we both fully and unconditionally forgave each other. I wasn't Pollyanna-ish enough to believe we could wipe the slate clean. I didn't fantasize that we could start over. Too much dirty water had flowed beneath the bridge for that to happen. And why would we want to anyway? We'd both come so far, learned so much over these past few painful years. We could only accept what had occurred in the past and make a conscious effort not to repeat the same mistakes, then begin from there.

"I really think we can have everything we want in life if we just throw all this hurt and anger away," I told Jerry one morning at breakfast as our cockatiels picked remnants of eggs and jelly off our plates. He didn't say anything at first, but I know he was listening by the way he nodded his head so slowly. I think he felt that sometimes he did all the talking for the two of us and he wanted to hear what I had to say.

"It almost feels like we've both carrying this big, heavy suitcase on our backs," I added. "God knows I'm tired of hauling that thing around."

Jerry got up from the table, walked over to me, and pretended to lift what appeared to be an imaginary suitcase off my back.

"You're right," he laughed. "The damn thing is heavy."

Most days now, I sit in my easy chair and stare out onto the vast, empty desert. I do my best to keep sane, positive thoughts in my mind. I think about how proud I am of my two boys, Stephen, who lives in Long Beach, California, and Peter, who lives in Flagstaff, Arizona. Both of them have evolved into happy, healthy, responsible adults. I think about my granddaughter, Skye, whom Stephen named in honor of my parents who helped raise him when I couldn't. And I try to coax the art and music to come back to me, to give me another chance.

I enjoy it here in this chair, looking out across the vastness of the parched desert, seeing things—like an approaching pickup or a coyote—a mile before it arrives outside our house. Seeing things this way makes me feel secure. It imbues my universe with a sense of predictability that it so seldom seems to possess. After Jerry disappears to go drive his cab, I often sit here for hours at a stretch, peering through my binoculars, studying the swirling tornado-like dust devils rising up from the desert floor, spinning furiously for a few minutes, then dying away into a faint brown smudge.

Sometimes I light up a cigarette, fill my lungs with smoke, then exhale, imagining that, besides smoke, I'm also blowing out all my memories. I love to watch them float and drift about the room like ghosts. I went off my medication again a few weeks back. I did it for no other reason than I was growing a bit bored with the new me. After all, being unbalanced can be truly exciting. You never know what's going to pop out of your head. When you're sane, however, you actually have to wait around for something interesting to happen before life ever turns fascinating. So far, though, I feel fine. The clarity is still there. Sometimes it's even blinding. Then again, there are days when the sky grows so dark I wonder if I'll ever see the sun again. Lately, I've been thinking a lot about Jerry and me. How much longer can two people like us hold on? It seems like everyone—myself included—wanted this to be one of those black-and-white love stories, the kind where two soul mates meet, fall in love, bliss happens, then a bit of tragedy tears them apart, yet they somehow manage to find their way back together and live happily ever after.

Jerry followed his heart when he decided to come back to me. Everyone around him was against it. Everyone assumed I was only going to cause him more pain. I hope that I don't. Because Jerry Newport is the first person, besides my sons, to love me unconditionally. He loved me for my good qualities and he seemed to see them in me when no one else could. Ours definitely isn't a black-and-white love story. It's one that constantly explodes with all the colors in the spectrum. It's brilliant, complex, and filled with the promise that real love truly does conquer all.

It may not cure autism. But for me it's been just what the doctor ordered for healing the human soul.

ACKNOWLEDGMENTS

My main reason for writing this book with Mary is that, between us, we offer over 108 years of experience combined. I want to give hope to people who have autism or Asperger's, as well as to those who parent and teach them. Beyond that, I want to give realistic hope to anyone who has ever felt so different that finding a partner seemed impossible. It is not impossible, but as we did, you have to learn to love yourself as you are and not as who you think the rest of the world wants you to be.

There is not enough space to thank all of the humans and other living creatures who have enriched my life. My highest order of thanks goes to my departed parents, Floyd and Loveda Newport, and to my brothers, John and Jim. From childhood, I thank my first real friend, the late Johnny Aichroth, and Islip classmates Steve Lazzaro, Don Shlimbaum, and John Veryzer for genuine friendship. I was also supported and inspired by many excellent teachers, especially music teacher Harvey Egan and English teacher Robert Cooper, both of whom must be teaching in heaven today.

From college, I thank my Delta Chi fraternity brothers, notably Mike Novak and Ken Brier, and Dr. Thomas F. Storer, retired math professor. My adult life was enriched by many friends from the taxi industry in San Diego—Steve Ferguson, the late Vic Burnett, and Michael J. Spadacini. San Diego City Councilman Floyd Morrow, Congressman Jim Bates, and candidate Phil Connor helped give me faith in working within the system.

I thank the late Donald Bremberg for his referrals, which led to jobs at Santa Monica Community College and later opportunities at UCLA. I'm thankful for the mentorship of supervisor Gail Chorna, aunt of an autistic boy, and Dr. Linda Demer, mother of two such boys. I survived two years at the Grant Elementary School Library, thanks to teachers Jackie Jaffe-Savage, Jan Baird, Mavis Smith, and Larry Doerflinger. I thank Dr. Linda Nickell for suggesting in 1989 that I see the movie *Rain Man,* which led to everything that followed. I thank Dr. Bernard Rimland for his good advice once that movie helped me make a personal connection.

From the parental world of autism-Aspergers, I learned better advocacy skills from the experience of Connie and Harvey Lapin, Tobey Arenberg, Anne Snowhook, and Charlene Wise. In fact, my first support group, AGUA, happened because of three visionary mothers, Kitty Rivet, Bunnie Guthrie, and the late Mary Preble. From that group, I still count many friends who have helped me in good and bad times, like Ken Brewer, Stephen Wise, Derrick Hall, Ilene Arenberg, Heidi Lissauer, and Johnathan Mitchell.

Finally, from Hollywood, I thank Robert Lawrence for his tireless dedication in helping Mary and me to share the fictionalized version of our story with many who need to hear it. Wayne Gilpin, head of Future Horizons publishing company, has been a friend as well as a mentor through two previous books and my initial attempts at public speaking.

I thank my fellow peer-writers Temple Grandin, Valerie Paradiz, Stephen Shore, and Liane Holliday Willey for their friendship and the inspiration that their excellent writing and advocacy provides. I thank Mike and Marie Bardach of Arizona, for helping me to get acquainted with a new city, Tucson, and for the many times they have bird-sat and dog-sat during my trips on behalf of autism and Asperger's syndrome.

I thank my terrific and tireless, ever accessible agent, Liza Dawson, for her guiding vision and for helping me find a cowriter, Johnny Dodd, whose experience and dedication were exceptional.

I thank Havis Dawson for his flexibility and accessibility as well. I thank my international agent, Chandler Crawford, for helping publishers all over the world to tell our story.

I thank Doris Cooper and Brett Valley at Simon & Schuster for their assistance. I hope those whose names are not mentioned will forgive me. My heart remains an open canvas, upon which you have all left permanent and positive strokes.

Jerry Newport
Arizona, 2006

Thanks to my boys—Peter and Steve, and to the staff at the Guidance Center of Flagstaff—Gina Robinson, Paul Ventura, Mike Depeche.

Mary Newport

Not a single word of this book would have been written without Liza Dawson, who guided this project from conception to delivery—you rock hard! To Big John and T-Lu, for teaching me the mysterious power of a well-crafted sentence. (An additional gracias to T-Lu for her exceptional proofreading.) To Diana, for the roller coaster—here's hoping you read this one. To Bruce McAllister, for his illuminating wisdom dispensed over phad thai and Singha. To Ron Arias, for his always open ears and insightful mind. To Liz Leonard, for just being so absolutely Liz Leonard! To Tom Fields-Meyer, for helping me glimpse a world I never understood until our talks. And to a cast of . . . well, dozens, who helped me pull this off while holding down a day job, especially Ron and Grace for their tireless tending of my progeny. To Priscilla Turner, for kicking over that first domino. To Diamond Joe Bruggeman, for his presence. To Rose, for her tireless, noble efforts at conquering gravity. To Doris Cooper, for cracking her editorial whip, and Brett Valley, for ensuring this project got finished. And special thanks to Jerry and Mary, for entrusting me with a story that has forever changed me.

Johnny Dodd